EARLY EJACULATION

Hidden Power

Easy book for masculine enhancement

Understand Study Act.

ANTONIO ALMA

or implied. Readers acknowledge that the author is not engaging in the rendering of legal, financial, medical or professional advice. The content within this book has been derived from various sources. Please consult a licensed professional before attempting any techniques outlined in this book.

By reading this document, the reader agrees that under no circumstances is the author responsible for any losses, direct or indirect, which are incurred as a result of the use of information contained within this document, including, but not limited to, — errors, omissions, or inaccuracies.

<u>**TABLE OF CONTENTS**</u>

Introduction

The whole world around us, the societies in which we mix. The civilizations that we have founded and destroyed. Interpersonal relationships, work, family, friends. The consideration of ourselves, the perception of us with respect to the world in which we live. Everything revolves around one thing. Sex. This emotion, this feeling so strong, that pushes us to the greatest madness. Sometimes controlling our lives as if we were puppets or as senseless animals living a life without meaning and with a single prerogative, give vent to this drive, as much as possible. Without there being a tomorrow.

But then, when the emotion has been released, a dull sad sound surrounds us, and we return to our life, to our routine that transports us in some absurd direction, ignoring that it is precisely from where we are going that we will do everything to return.

The struggles with schoolmates to prove who was the strongest, the scooter in high school to look independent, the car at 18 years old to make it clear that you were already one of the greats. Then the job, to look for the best paid, the best paid and prove that you could afford everything you wanted. The gym, to seem stronger and more athletic. The examples are endless and you know most of them too. And why all this? To have her, the woman who makes your heart beat, to show that you are an Alpha man, a man to choose from, a man to marry. But above all, a man to desire and to make love to us.

Now you have a house, a good job well paid, maybe a company, you go three times a week to the gym, you go around the city with a nice custom, a nice important car, you're full of interesting commitments and finally the women start to get curious about you.

You have everything you could want materially, but what happens, after only a few short periods of time since your relationship began, the emotional compromise that you have with her begins to tilt. She doesn't look at you as she did at the beginning, she doesn't call you so often, she doesn't wait for you at night to kiss you when you get home. Already all the superfluous starts to crumble, and you stay with that feeling of sadness. You know what the problem is, you know what the missing piece in this puzzle is. Now you just have to decide whether to admit it and become aware of it, or pretend that the situation is not up to you. You can find a thousand kinds of excuses not to deal with the problem, there is always a way to pass the responsibility on to others. That's what 40% of men do...

But you're different. If you are reading this book, it is because you have realized that maybe there is a problem, but you have not surrendered to the condition in which you find yourself, you are looking for a solution. You are convinced that there is, and I am here to show you that you are right.

There has been a gradual reduction in the virility of men, and this can be attributed to poor eating habits, inactivity, or extreme exercising. They no longer have the energy required to give a full performance in bed. For some of these men, they cannot get a full erection, and they experience erectile dysfunction. For others, they get a full erection but prematurely ejaculate, as they find it difficult to perform for a significant period of time. These groups possibly include a higher number of people than those who do not get an erection at all.

If you are reading this book, you might be familiar with the experience of frequent early ejaculation, bringing possible discomfort to you and your partner. No doubt, it can be infuriating. You feel humiliated, your wounded pride may make you feel uncomfortable, and you start to feel like you haven't pleasured your partner. However, is this problem real?

As annoying as it can be, cumming early a few times is normal. Most guys experience this, so there is usually no need to be worried. But what if you constantly experience early ejaculation? What happens if sex ends after only one minute, or occasionally after just a few seconds? What if the thought of sex makes you consistently feel agitated, embarrassed and distraught because you know you are unable to last? What if this is how it has always been for you?

If you can relate with all these, it is possible you are experiencing premature ejaculation (PE). This is the most prevalent type of sexual dysfunction experienced by men. According to research, about 30 percent of men suffer from premature ejaculation, but despite its prevalence, it might be impossible to recognize this by speaking to your friends.

Saying that it is hard to speak about PE is an understatement. It is difficult for most guys to own up to any type of sexual issue, particularly an issue as delicate as PE. Stereotypical depictions of premature ejaculation in movies like "Fast Times at Ridgemont High" and "American Pie" has helped spread the wrong belief that premature ejaculation is only experienced by horny teenagers or selfish men.

In reality, anyone can experience premature ejaculation, regardless of age, knowledge about sex, or even experience with sex. Although there are effective drugs for treating erectile dysfunction; sadly, there are no effective drugs for treating premature ejaculation directly.

This book primarily concerned with premature ejaculation and discusses natural and effective treatments of this problem. The techniques recommended in this book are simple and highly effective. In my opinion, natural techniques are the best way of treating these issues, which we will discuss in detail.

I belong to the school of thought that self-help books should be precise, direct and made of only relevant information. It should not be filled with redundant details. Recommended methods should be effective and simple to follow. This book was written with consideration of these principles.

The exercise section discusses how exercises can help to develop the muscles used for ejaculation. Engaging in these exercises regularly can help one to achieve healthy ejaculation in just one month.

Ten simple and effective yoga techniques are also discussed. The efficiency of these yoga techniques is high. The chapter also includes a few tricks and tips that can be used while transitioning to the stage of no premature ejaculation.

I am here to assure you that it is simple for anyone to overcome premature ejaculation and experience a pleasurable and normal sexual life.

Chapter 1:

Today's Expectations and Realities About Sex

Coping as a man can be difficult. Whether you live in the evolved Western world or anywhere else, it is likely that you are programmed to think that being a man is all about establishing your life, acquiring certifications, and attaining success. A strong drive is ingrained in us to always aim for the best and achieve the best results in our lives and that of others. We are taught to aim for excellence, personally and professionally, and failure to do this results in thoughts of ourselves as 'disappointments,' 'underachievers,' or 'losers.'

Paradoxically, it is impossible to be perfect; so, is there any point in pursuing something that is not attainable? Worse still, why should you introduce this ideology into the aspects of your life that are supposed to be all about being satisfied, care-free and joyful? As you might have suspected, your sex life is an example of that aspect; here, you should forget about your "responsibility to accomplish" and concerns about "being successful."

Your narcissistic behaviors should be curbed when it comes to sex; ideally, your goals should not be centered on performance, ways of being perfect in bed, or proving to your partner that you can make them orgasm from penetration. You should aim towards selecting a fulfilling method of lovemaking such that you and your partner both derive pleasure.

Come to terms with the fact that you are not a sex robot, but a man who is capable of giving and taking pleasure during sex. Instead of being concerned with achieving orgasms and arousal, sex and sexuality are better approached with satisfaction and pleasure in mind. The degree of pleasure and satisfaction is purely mental, so by learning to broaden your vision in this field, it will also increase your level of perception of sex.

Hints of sacred and spiritual sex

In nature, man is biologically designed to come in the shortest possible time, unlike a woman who has been designed to last as long as possible.
Why?
To safeguard the possibility of procreation.
We are now far from those times, but in the animal kingdom still lives the same priority. That is, to procreate and keep one's life safe. When we were in the jungle or when we lived in the forests, the threats to our safety were enormous and continuous. There was no time for foreplay, hugs, caresses. For the human being, the only main thing was to fertilize our female, to indulge our instincts for a moment and hope that for those few moments of vulnerability, nobody would attack us.

So, **first of all**, premature ejaculation is not a synonym that you are wrong, on the contrary, you are perfectly in line with your primordial nature. The problem is that it would be better to adapt with what are the circumstances of today's society. Don't worry, it's simpler than they make it seem. Let's move on...

With the passing of time, man has evolved, discovering more and more deeply the world around him, including himself. We discovered solar energy, electrical energy, atomic energy...and included, an equally powerful and fundamental energy, that is, SEXUAL ENERGY. I am convinced that this is the energy that dominates our world today even if we are using it sadly, in the worst of ways.

Our body thinks and organizes itself according to priorities.

Yes, the production of our sperm takes away almost 30% of the total we have available to live our days as men. The average time it takes our bodies to fill 100% of our sperm supply is 5 days. These data are based on a person of about 30-35 years.
Every time we ejaculate we are taking energy away from our vital centers such as brain, pancreas, liver, lungs, intestine, Pineal gland, thyroid, etc..

Once ejaculated the first priority of our body, after breathing, will be to return to produce sperm. In doing so, our metabolism, whether we want it or not, will direct 30% of the energy available in this laborious matter. So I would give up the question that says ... Why do I fall asleep every time I finish making love? But let's go a little deeper.
The average man tends to masturbate in life, more or less, once a day. Do you know what this means? Do you realize what it means?
80% of people on earth have lived, live and will live most of their lives at 30% less than their chance.

When I realized this, I remained petrified. Only the idea of bringing my hands closer to my intimate area made me feel more tired.
I believe that now you will think twice about coming to your next love meeting. The curious thing is that if by chance I came into it, this spectacular and great energy that we possess and produce, would thus be donated free of charge to its recipient! What if it was you and you kept this miraculous energy? Just try to imagine a slow, long, passionate emotional relationship, but why not, even the hard, strong

and animal sex of a single night where in the end, instead of
falling exhausted in the blankets, you get up leaving her body
exhausted on the mattress. It's not fiction, it's not fantasy. It's
reality, and I'm here for you to realize it.
Word of an early Ex-ejaculator.

So, **point number 2**, don't think that your seed is just a
liquid that you have there to make children.
It's something extremely precious for your physical health,
think about it before giving it to the first stranger that
happens!

There are many advantages to be gained from not ejaculating.
As I said before, this non-dispersion of energy allows the
body to use it and redirect it to where it is most needed. This
example should clarify the concept I want to express: imagine
you've been a hardened smoker for more than 15 years. At
one point, for various regions, you decided to stop smoking.
Surely you will encounter difficulties at first, especially
mental ones. In addition to nicotine addiction, one of the
main reasons why people can't quit is because they can't give
up their acquired habits (the same goes for ejaculation). Let's
assume that you did it in this case. Imagine how you would
feel to live your days with 100% of your lungs! I'll tell you,
you'll feel like flying a meter from the ground.
I'm telling you, you're gonna feel like you're gonna be flying a
foot above the ground.
In addition, this accumulated energy is like making you a
super-charged magnet for the other sex. Women, even if
unconsciously, feel the vibration of this testosterone stored in
your body, and are attracted to it. As the days go by, and as
you continue to keep this fantastic energy within you, you
will notice the change in the way they look at you. For
example, at work colleagues, at the supermarket unknown

women, when you go out on the street with friends or dying,
etc.. You will become more fascinating if you can explain,
more seductive, more attractive. And all this will also
considerably improve your self-esteem.
In case you have a wife or a moron, the effect will still be
beneficial. Living together, unknowingly, she will notice this
vibration coming from your body, increasing and
maintaining her desire for you.

Sexual Skill vs. Sexual Performance

Wanting to improve yourself to become a better lover is different from forcing yourself to become one. Having the desire to enhance your sex life is normal; but if you are overburdened with performing perfectly and thinking of premature ejaculation as the worst thing to happen, simply expect to achieve the opposite results. With this thinking you could experience performance fright, a feeling that is based on the misconception that you MUST be exceptional in bed, and you very well might lose your desire and natural inclination to have sex altogether.

Your natural desire to improve your sexual skills is totally unrelated to this mentality. As a man, you should not have to aim for performance; instead, aim for pleasure. Making love with an attractive woman whom you have artfully seduced mainly involves pleasure, and not obligations or duties. Confirm from any woman you like and expect to hear this exactly: if you enjoy, she probably will too. But if you make it a duty to give her pleasure then it will be impossible for either of you to truly enjoy.

One common misconception of sex is that it should be fast, mechanical, and perfectly effortless. Practice helps to develop a skill. For instance, when you first learned to ride a bike, the constant practice helped you adapt and learn how to remain stable on the bike. Sex for the purpose of procreation is quite easy; however, if you would like to experience joy, satisfaction, and sexual confidence while creating a solid sexual relationship with your lover, then you have to treat it like any other skill and learn to practice it. In perfecting this skill, you need to be consistent using the exercises and tips in this book.

A common misconception is that having sex should take

hours. After being handled for so long, the woman might eventually become tired. A lot of women experience extreme discomfort after a while and they might ask you if you are about to cum. This could be annoying for the both of you.

Another myth is that the man is entirely responsible for spectacular sex. I would like to know, how many times have you gotten a less-than-satisfying blowjob from a woman? How many times have you been fully erect in her mouth only for your boner to deflate almost immediately after she scrapes the tip of your penis with her teeth? Perhaps, you can vividly recall that time you told a woman to rub your cock and somehow she misinterpreted this as pulling it off completely.

No lover is perfect, man or woman. Just as you don't cast blame on a woman's 'mistakes,' also try to give yourself the same compassion.

Another misconception is that sex is a one-man thing wrong. The woman can support a major part of your learning process in controlling your excitement and determining the quality of sex you have. Two heads are better than one. You have to set aside 20-30 minutes for foreplay to help you adjust to your body's emotional and physical signals. By doing this, you will have enough time to understand and take note of your body's signs of sexual arousal.

You will have the ability to try out the techniques you will be learning during arousal at your own preferred pace. Ultimately, there should be adequate time for you to practice and adapt to controlling even higher degrees of arousal in situations that are simpler than those involving penetration.

To reduce the level of your arousal during foreplay, avoid the point of no return, and try not to stimulate your penis. Your muscles have to be relaxed and breathe from within. We will discuss this method in detail later in this book. What am I referring to as foreplay? I am talking about sexual massage, not the usual sleepy massage. Foreplay massage is when you are rubbing and stimulating her erogenous and non-erogenous zones.

Know that your brain is the most significant sex organ in your body. In the course of the exercise, you have to be conscious of your thoughts. You must be aware of what your mind concentrates on. The most beneficial thing here is to think positively and with great optimism. If you concentrate on exercise one at a time, you will achieve exceptional success. Learning how to focus your attention and train your mind is very important and ample time will be devoted to this topic later on.

Regard sex positively. Sex is enjoyable. The pleasure derived is enjoyable too. Suppressing your joy to control ejaculation is unnecessary. Be personally responsible for the development of your sexual skills. Do these exercises diligently. GIVING UP IS NOT AN OPTION. Additionally, you have to find a stable ground between understanding the techniques I will be teaching and expressing them in your own way.

Get ready to relax. One of the first things we will learn later on is how to relax using specific relaxation techniques. While doing that, you will understand how to adapt, persevere, and contribute when it comes to your sexual relationships.

The Role of Pornography

It is true that pornography might destroy one's sexual life, but how and to what extent is still debated by specialists. Porn is considered an awful guideline for sex. This is mainly because the acts are unreal, the movies have been edited, the actors are experts, and these movies are often provided for male enjoyment. Porn makes sex look automatic and spontaneous, void of feelings or emotions, which is not the reality of it.

Depending on sex as an excitant could be very dangerous to your sexual life. This may result in the emulation of bad sexual habits, such as very fast sex movements. This could have a huge effect on your orgasm. Also, a sexual life developed from porn will lack intimacy, which many women and men crave.

It is also very important to state that porn has a way of training our brains to be highly sensitive and respond to an overload of sexual stimuli. Our brains overload by secreting more endorphins than normal. As time goes on, our brains become less sensitive to this overload of sexual stimuli and then require a much higher stimulus in order to be aroused. As a result of this, a porn user might progress to more hardcore porn.

It would be nice to put some heart and humanity into this pornographic commercial industry that stereotypes sex, people and sometimes becomes the only way to learn to become good lovers. It is not to demonise porn, it is to make people think.
We know that at an intellectual level porn is a fantasy, but the mind (also proven by science) does not distinguish between what is real and what is fiction. This also includes what we see on the monitor.

The main point is that we live in a hyper-sexualized society, continuous sexual stimuli on TV and in billboards.
In man, in addition to a loss of energy through the loss of sperm, it mainly diverts attention from the body, sexual energy is not a mental energy, it is an electrical energy that flows into the bowels of the nervous system, muscles, etc..

Pornographic videos nourish and feed only new fantasies, instead of nourishing the higher vital centers such as the heart and brain. They develop an inability to stay in the present moment with the partner to feel the energy flowing in the body because the visual stimulation is very strong for us men and these images are recorded in our minds and we want to realize them by distracting us from flowing in the moment. Also, as men, we tend to imitate, and porn is sadly perhaps the only source from which we can learn about sex in this society. Other sources on sexuality are mostly anatomy and courses on sexually transmitted diseases.

The objectification of the woman is around the corner; in porn, the performance anxiety it produces in young people is enormous, and the high standards do not allow us to feel how we would really like to make love. We become standardised and above all mechanical.
For this reason, here, the curiosity to know, saves the most 'daring!

A good sexual education would lead to the knowledge that ejaculation is not an orgasm but only a consequence of it.
True and lasting pleasure is a place to which we can have access together with our partner developing a good intimacy and connection first of all with ourselves and with our body.

Today porn is a loss of energy, but with ejaculation allows the man to relax or better to lose energy and then relax because exhausted.

Porn is a poor, heartless imitation of sexual intercourse.

Energy can be used in various ways to get to know one another and open up altered states of consciousness and it is possible to channel it into our lives to live a life closer to our body, more authentic.

Today the risk is that two people who watch porn videos, when they meet in the bedroom, know or believe how to give pleasure to the other and neither is really able to. Since ancient times, sex has been the way to evolve and enter realms and universes that through "little death" we can probe and connect with the source.

Porn simplifies the man's sexuality, objectifies the woman and consequently the human being. without leaving room for the heart, to live this experience that can become sacred.

I believe that adults and young people have the right to know the potential of sex.
Let us not demonize porn, but let us not diminish the psychological conditioning that subtly alienates us from the beauty of sexuality.
Let us not demonize porn, but let us not diminish the psychological conditioning that subtly alienates us from the beauty of sexuality.

Premature Ejaculation

The most common type of sexual dysfunction experienced by men is premature ejaculation; however, it is somehow still one of the least understood. Like I said previously, most of us must have experienced early ejaculation at one time or the other. This can be annoying, but if you constantly ejaculate too quickly, you might be suffering from PE. To know more about premature ejaculation you must first understand the physiology behind ejaculation.

You might think that ejaculation, the discharge of seminal fluid from your body, is restricted to your testicles, penis and other sex organs. This is incorrect. Actually, the nervous system controls the majority of the functions. The nervous system is composed of the sympathetic nervous system (SNS) and the parasympathetic nervous system (PNS).

The SNS controls your body's "flight or fight" response, which comes into play when you are tense. This helped the early man to evade or fight aggressive predators. Nowadays, your flight or fight response can be deployed in less dangerous situations, such as when you have a big meeting coming up. The PNS, on the other hand, controls your body's "rest and digest" response. This is characterized by a decreased heart rate, reduced blood pressure and other processes synonymous with relaxation.

Sexual arousal is the first step in the process leading up to premature ejaculation. It usually starts with direct excitation of your penis through oral sex, touching, massaging, or even sex. A response by your brain through signals is sent to the spinal cord. Your parasympathetic nervous system then makes your penis erect. Due to this, there is a rhythmic contraction in the muscles in your seminal vesicles, prostate gland (both of which function in the production of seminal fluid) and vas deferens (the tube that forms a connection between the urethra and testicles). This then causes a movement of semen out of your body through the urethra and these glands. The sympathetic nervous system controls this process.

While ejaculating, you experience a sensation of intense pleasure. This is known as an 'orgasm.' When this process constantly happens sooner than you or your partner wants, it is then considered premature ejaculation. There are conflicting definitions of premature ejaculation in the medical community, and as such, there is no clear definition of exactly how premature the ejaculation must be to be considered PE. However, the most recent and frequently used definition by the International Society of Sexual Medicine (ISSM) defines premature ejaculation as "a male sexual dysfunction indicated by ejaculation that invariably or almost invariably happens before or within one minute of vaginal penetration; and has a negative individual outcomes such as anxiety, discomfort, discontent and/or the reluctance to engage in sexual activity" (ISSM, 2019).

Though additional research is required, some studies estimate that 30 percent of men experience premature ejaculation at a point in their lifetime. In my opinion, more than 30 percent of men, particularly those below 40 are struggling with PE. If we look at the embarrassment, humiliation, and hesitation of men identifying with premature ejaculation and the large proportion of women who would rather fake an orgasm than allow their partner to feel humiliated or like a sexual novice, coupled with the fact that there is an age-long disagreement on the definition of premature ejaculation, we can safely conclude that we have uncovered very little on the full effect of premature ejaculation on men and their partners.

Women's Top Five Misconceptions About Premature Ejaculation

It is understandable why females might not be able to relate to PE. Since they do get to brinks of imminent orgasms in the same way as males, it is hard for them to picture having no control over climax in the same way. This combined with the unwillingness of men to open up about their sexual performance (or non-performance as it is), the female folk, in a bid to understand the whole thing, come up with theories of their own. Below are five universal fallacies women hold about PE:

PE indicates enthusiasm and ecstasy

A lot of women tend to feel all buttered up at the sight of your PE. They assume that they are so enticing that you can't restrain yourself. It may seem easier to let them run with that falsehood in order to make her feel good about herself, also helping you escape having to explain your predicament. This easy way out is as wrong as letting her think that if you suffered from erectile dysfunction your condition was because of her too (which certainly will *not* stroke her ego). A majority of men with problems with sexual performance don't have their spouse or partner to blame for their dysfunction. Thus, no matter how tempted you are about letting her ride on that horse of falsehood—don't do it

You're not attracted to her

You can't help if you're not particularly interested in her. But this usually isn't the case. A terrible misconception is when the woman concludes that you are just not attracted to her if you aren't having sex regularly. In fear of being discovered, men with PE might try to avoid sex by coming up with flimsy excuses every time or refuse to go beyond foreplay (if they are even bold enough to engage in foreplay). This leaves the woman feeling unwanted and unattractive. All the while, you know that you are hiding something from her and sooner rather than later, she will find out. This deception only makes the situation worse and hurts your relationship miserably. Unfortunately, some men would rather avoid the truth and destroy a relationship than come clean about their PE.

You are greedy and self-centered in bed

Contrary to the popular misconception, men with PE are usually extremely considerate about their sexual performance and if they have satisfied their partner. Unfortunately, many women don't understand this. Every time the man climaxes before the woman even begins, she begins to see herself as being used by the man. We can refer back to Lorena Bobbitt. After confessing to chopping the penis off of her husband, John Wayne Bobbitt, she was quoted to have said, "he never waits for me," referring to what she believed was her partner's self-centeredness. Of course we are not certain why he never waited, but what if he had PE? Then instead of the self-centered behavior assumed of him, he might have, to the contrary, been extremely sensitive and concerned about his wife's pleasure.

You are unskilled and a rookie

Naivety about premature ejaculation may make the woman

erroneously translate it to ineptitude. But it really is not their fault, especially when people don't really talk about it—*the truth about it*. Her only knowledge about PE may be what she has heard fellow women joke about or from something she saw in a movie. Unfortunately, these images she has garnered from unverifiable sources give her the impression that only oversexed and randy teenage boys get PE. We are beginning to learn this is far from the case. Men suffering from PE could very well be skilled and sensitive to his partner's desires. Though unfortunately, they are incapable of turning their well-meaning objectives into actualizations.

You are dull and boring sexually

Over time, men suffering from PE create a routine they follow to prolong their erections for as long as possible. It does help them, but to an unsuspecting partner sex with you becomes drab and monotonous. Let me repeat myself: your brain is your most essential sexual tool. Try to create a fantasy with your partner, even if it is just talking, which will still bring an edge to your sex life. We will discuss more visualization technique later on.

Don't forget that naivety, oblivion, and lore's about PE are the bedrock of these misconceptions. The good news is that telling your partner about this book and encouraging her to also be well informed can correct these fallacies. Even more important is coming clean to her about your condition. It could save your relationship.

<h1 style="text-align:center">Chapter 2:</h1>

Causes of Premature Ejaculation

There are different reasons for the individual variations in premature ejaculation. The majority of the premature ejaculation cases do not present symptoms. If you occasionally experience premature ejaculation, it will be beneficial to assess if these symptoms are also noticed.

The Desire to Cum

I want to be as explicit as possible here. When we are sexually excited, an internal conviction just tells you to let loose. I call this the "desire to cum." I used to mentally justify the reasons why I should just offload and at that particular time, it seemed logical to me. This decision was one I usually regretted.

It is logically valid to say that you cum too fast because of your desire to cum. We all experience the uncontrollable impulse to cum, right? This is definitely true. And for a fraction of a second, I would not condemn this desire. Our life's journey revolves around that itch to search for pleasure. As true descendants of god and goddesses, continue that. The uncontrollable impulse to cum is a physiological process that supersedes your decision to choose what happens. But it is important to consider the context with which we are discussing our orgasms. You need to think about your partner's orgasms, your own, and your sexual satisfaction as a whole.

In the next chapters you will learn the concept of "percentage of excitement", a concept that you will have to study, practice and train. The main focus that you will approach through the exercises described below is Listening to Yourself. Only by learning to listen to yourself, to feel how you feel, and by observing what is happening inside your body, will you learn to control it.

Overwhelming Excitement

This is a relatively common occurrence; and like me, a lot of people must have experienced it at least once. You are totally attracted to that sex-on-wheels who also happens to be attracted to you. This turns you on so much that before you are even aware, your shorts or even her skirt is filled with cum. My goodness! Recalling those humiliating times is something I truly hate, but if I wasn't sure that this issue could be solved for you in no time, I wouldn't have brought back those sticky memories.

Experiencing intense excitement is synonymous with being a warm-blooded and virile man. The level of excitability decreases with age, so it is highest in young people. It is normal when young men who are new to sex find it difficult to control their response for the first few times. As this is the only way we have been taught, we are irrationally led by the internal wave surging within us. A large number of us are unaware that there is another method of handling this energy overload. If you persevere and you are ready to hold back for a decade or two, excitability decreases as you become older so that might work. It is normal when young people who are new to sex find it difficult to control their response for the first time. It is the same example as before, that of the bicycle, which repeats itself. The first time we mount a bike, we have to learn to realize, the space, the balance, the speed and all in a position that we normally do not have the habit of mastering. Result? We fall!

In the same way, in our first sexual relations, we are irrationally guided by the internal wave that rises inside us. There's her, there's us, two naked bodies, maybe it's the first time. There is contact, you don't know where to put your hands or maybe you would like to put them everywhere. We are used to touching ourselves, of course, but touching the body of another person and different. There is fear, frenzy, the heart beats madly, you sweat and you feel cold at the same time. Oh, my God, I'm tough, you might wonder if it's time to go in. You touch her, her vagina, and you don't understand. Then try to rest the tip of your penis. Oh, my God, but where's the entrance, maybe you're there. Yes, I am inside. I did it. Mom, that's nice. That's great. Oooh, it's so soft, enveloping, warm. But, but... what's going on? No, no, fuck, no, I'm coming. No, I came.

Some time ago I stopped to reflect on a cartoon found by chance in a newspaper. It was very stimulating. There was a boy sitting in front of a piano, I believe in the attempt to play it. A man was drawn behind him, looking at him. The man said to the boy, "let it go, you're not capable!" and the boy at the piano replied, "if I leave it alone, I'll never be capable! This I think is a concept that we can apply to anything that interests us in life.

Never giving up is the key, so read on.

Worry and Tension

I hope I can trust you with this secret, but the key to becoming a master at ejaculation is relaxation. A lot of things can cause worry and stress when it comes to sex. I am quite amazed at how many men blow this reality off too quickly. These are some of the common stressors responsible for cumming quickly:

- Putting in an effort not to cum

- Relationship problems

- Lack of self-confidence

- Time pressure

- Illness or weakness

- Religious beliefs that sex is unclean, sinful, or bad

- Fear of sexually transmitted diseases (STDs) and pregnancy

- Worries about being discovered

- Fear of underperforming (am I skilled enough to satisfy my lover?)

The first reason seems unbelievable. Trying not to think about cumming can make you cum too early. However contradictory this sounds, it's the truth.

Conditioning to Go Fast

According to sex therapists, quick climax starts as a youth and then develops to become an automatic reflex that continues later in life. While growing up, most of us were scared about getting caught having sex. If you can recall, most of our sexual adventures involved doing a quick one in the back seat of our dad's car, or on the sofa in the living room, finishing just in time as to not get caught by anybody who might pop up soon. Our thoughts were so centered on not getting caught that sex was too quick and unfulfilling.

Do you remember your first real lover, your hand? Personally, I preferred my right hand. Masturbation for a fast release was the best way of making it less likely to be discovered. Men are wired to think that it is better not to be discovered while masturbating, for various reasons. To get satisfaction, and eventual release, this was usually done covertly and fast. Additionally, it creates a particular habit of strain within the body regarding sexual issues and this forms the basis for subsequent sexual experiences. It starts with men masturbating and cumming very fast on their beds, or in the shower, hoping that they would not be discovered. Then it progresses to having sex with their girlfriends in their room, or even in the back seat of their car, yet, hoping not to be discovered too. And this continues throughout their life, and marriage, unaware that there are other better ways.

That's how it works. For many of us, the approach to sexuality is intimately linked to unnecessary emotions such as fear, anxiety, shame. What was eventually meant to be an experience of joy and discovery is thus transformed into an unconscious trauma that we carry with us for the rest of our lives.

What I'm saying is this. If you want to masturbate, do it. Don't think it's immoral. Don't feel guilty because of your religion. Don't believe that you are committing a sin. If it really was something wrong to masturbate, surely God, would not have made your hands come right up to your inner zone! Think about it!
This does not mean that I want to push you into masturbation in an uncontrolled way, I recommend it. But when that sense comes, that irrepressible libido, that desire you can't resist, you organize to make your experience something unique.
How? That said, I did. Keep reading.

Check it out and make sure no one comes to disturb you. Take some time, even an hour, why not. Search and select a safe and secure environment. You could also use music, I sometimes do it. Don't rush to watch porn, wait. Strip down, and maybe start moving around your room naked and sensually to the rhythm of music. Don't bring your hands directly on your penis, wait. Allow yourself to be caressed, explore your body, give yourself affection and love. Your body is in constant collaboration with your life, show it that you are grateful. Without haste you can start to touch yourself, but I recommend you to try even more than one position. Yes, let yourself be indulged. Without haste, because no one is running after you. Use your imagination, try to visualize the images that could excite you the most and not the ones that a porn gives you. Explore your mind and its hiding places. Breathe deeply, inhale the vibration you are emitting, enjoy it, stay in the present, enjoy the present. Create ups and downs of excitement, find out how close you can get to the point of No Return. There is no fixed time, don't think about time. Give voice to this moment, laugh if you feel like laughing, shout or anxious if you feel like doing it. Don't be

ashamed. Then, when you feel ready, come. But when this moment comes, put all your passion into it. Don't leave anything out. Listen to how the vibrations of your body change. Feel and live this moment of release. Now wait. Don't rush to clean yourself. You're not dirty. Keep massaging yourself. Give yourself a few more minutes of pleasure. Allow your heart to slowly return to normal pulsations.
Now yes, congratulations on the trip, welcome home.

Purpose of Orgasm

Our lives in the world today revolve around standards, purpose, and living up to expectations. What is the stereotypical standard of performance for the perfect virile man? That perfect man is so familiar with women that he is capable of satisfying anyone of them. He expertly handles each of them until they crumble and yield to their desire. Until they are totally wild with passion, he is quiet, and powerful as well. Then with an aggressive release, showing that they have never had better, he experiences a high-intensity orgasm at the same time as his partner. Truth be told, the Big O (a high-intensity orgasm) is what our backward and sexually restrained society compares us with. We were taught that the goal of sex is to release all your accumulated sexual energy with the highest intensity of orgasm. Most times, we are caught in the web of our partner's similar conviction fueled by extended periods of sexual dissatisfaction. As incredible as that could feel, you would be amazed to know the importance of other things such as care, cuddling, and affection, to a typical woman mean the world. One study I read recently estimated that most women prefer intimacy to sex (Smalley, 2018). We are wired to hurry at breakneck speed into orgasm. While hurrying, we do not enjoy the emotions and sensations involved. In the Western world, sex is believed to be a dash to the climax that is followed by the physical exhaustion of lovers. The Ultimate Ecstatic Solution is closely related to the eastern perspective regarding physical love, where lovers gradually climb greater heights of bliss over and over again. And this is what we aim to master using Tantra.

But what is Tantra? I should probably answer this question by writing another book.

Tantra is the Secret, it is the unknown way to happiness, it is loss and rebirth. Tantra is everything around us. In short, in order not to go on for too long and to give an idea also to those who hear this term for the first time in their lives, Tantra is a set of techniques that we use to enter into ourselves, to approach our most authentic Self and to dismantle the illusion in which we have imprisoned ourselves. Tantra is the source of pure Love. This pure Love is us, so we are the source because we come from it. Tantra is a discipline that teaches us to return to the source, to return to our true IO.

The Mind

The mind is undoubtedly a strong sex organ. Dr. Andrew Harrison, who is also a well-known Tantra teacher in California, believes that "energy flows in the same direction as attention." Concentrate on pleasure and you experience deeper emotions. Try not to cum, and you will still find yourself cumming.

We attract what we concentrate on. For instance, if your entire focus is centered on your genitals, then all your sexual energy is directed to that 'tiny' hole in your 'tiny' head. If you are focused on helping your partner orgasm, chances are that you will experience one soon. There are numerous case studies purporting the psychological causes of premature ejaculation. Focusing on pleasuring your partner is the main stimulating solution that helps you derive additional pleasure from sex while controlling your ejaculation.

The illusions of the mind, which are permeating mental pictures or goals you are completely focused on, distract you from fully concentrating on what is happening presently. Is it possible for you to genuinely appreciate what is presently going on with all these overwhelming mental distractions? Rather than this, you have to redirect your attention to your senses, your entire body, sensations, and emotions—all the possible avenues of pleasure. We will be discussing this subsequently.

The purpose of training the mind is to move out of your head and move into your body. Be still and focus on the moment, focus on those incredible sensations exuding from your pleasure zones. Let go of all your standards and expectations. Just go with the flow. Avoid overexerting yourself or your lover just for the Big O. Learning to flow with your sexual energy without trying to control the result will help you ride the wave in a natural and relaxed manner.

Separate, Not Joint Experience

In the world today, sex is sometimes regarded as a secret because it is forbidden to discuss it. Our insecurities are concealed as we crack offensive jokes and do not discuss it in public. Many of us are consumed with the thought of making the first move, or how to start with a long-term partner rather than reveling in the enjoyable moment of foreplay. And this might account for why a lot of us accumulate those strains and tensions that we discussed earlier which are responsible for premature ejaculation.

We are not taught that sex is an intimate connection between souls communicating their primal nature through the revered gifts of bodies. Only some of us learn the skillful harmonization of these instruments to create exceptional pleasure. How do we learn that sex is a transfer of energy between living beings who desire to give and take pleasure? When you are wanted and accepted as you are with no expectations concerning your performance, then you can just chill and allow nature to play its part in your sexual lives.

This is one of the reasons why bonding with your partner is required for the Main Stimulating Solution. This refers to understanding your needs and responses, having honest discussions concerning them, respecting those of your partner, and engaging as equals. Rather than 'screwing' your partner, you have to engage in activities like sharing. Really, you don't have to gag, you're in a position to allow room for changes, pal. You started this journey because you seek a change, right?

Just so you know, all the techniques in the Main Stimulating Solution are totally effective for both sexes. Tantra involves yin and yang vibes, which we usually correlate with the female and male sex. However, experts have discovered that everyone possesses both vibes within and adequate practice can help us act on both. I have put in the effort to make the language as acceptable as possible to lesbian and gay partners but I might not be doing this well. So kindly accept this disclaimer that everything here is effective and involves you as well. In reality, Subtle Energy eXchange (S.E.X.) is possibly more applicable to same-sex partners.

There are variations in sexual responses among partners. Although most women require a lot of stimulation, some are able to cum very fast. They like being touched all over their body. If touched too intimately, then they are done. So, who ensures that each partner derives maximum pleasure? The complete responsibility is shared between the two partners. Being partners involves communicating your needs and respecting those of your partners. If we deviate from this, we create the condition that results in strain, tension, and anxiety—a sure fire way to spraying your seed suddenly.

If you are not in a relationship and you are looking for a partner to sexually satisfy, this entire idea of sex as a connection might be harder than finding someone prepared to merely play in the sack. It's a joke to think that you can solely satisfy any woman without her participation. Get rid of the notion that the satisfaction of your partner is your exclusive duty. This is a partnership and a lot of women like it that way.

I imagine the woman as a pot full of water where after we should cook the pasta! We are the flame that heats the pot.

In most cases, man tends to give a great initial impulse to this flame. A large blast of heat embraces the pot from underneath, considerably increasing the temperature of the metal on which it is heated. But you have a few minutes the flame runs out. The result is that the temperature of the water has remained unchanged, or at most it has only risen a few degrees. Once again, damn rush. Even today, no pasta! Do you really want to cook, do you really want to eat a succulent dish? Eliminate any hurry and take your time. With elegance and ease, get into the kitchen. Turn around, maybe open a bottle of wine in the meantime. Enjoy this moment where you decided to cook. Light the fire and put the flame to a minimum. Watch as the water gets warmer, watch as the first bubbles begin to form and the steam begins to release into the air.

You understand, once the water is boiling, you even have the possibility to turn off the flame for a few minutes, it will not be a problem. The pot will still remain at the temperature, and when you feel ready, just return to light the flame, and you can continue to cook.

Now all I have to do is wish you luck: Enjoy your meal.

Prostatitis

The prostate gland is an important sex organ as it is a part of the initial discharge stage of ejaculation. Inflammation or increase in the size of the prostate gland is known as 'prostatitis' and it can increase your sensitivity to stimulation causing you to cum very fast. If you are finding it difficult to pee or you are feeling sensitive there, consult your doctor so that you can be referred to a urologist for proper examination. If you are on any prescription medications, discuss the possible side effects.

Luckily, there are a few natural solutions to enhance your prostate health. Peyum and Saw Palmetto are my personal favorites. They are readily available at the health store. Studies have discovered that these supplements can be very beneficial for your prostate. I always hear about new natural solutions and love to try them out.

There are a few other common substances that can cause an inflammation of your prostate and increase your sensitivity to cumming. Take a wild guess. If you drink alcohol and coffee or smoke, it is advisable for you to stay away from them in the course of this program. Trust me, I am far from being a moralist trying to make you stop your bad habits. I have tried out almost everything and I am a firm believer of anything that gives pleasure. My warnings to you concerning irritation of your prostate are simply a medical fact. Smoking and alcohol are the major causes of most erection problems in men (Godman, 2019). Other recreational and prescription drugs can significantly affect your sexual health too. The Main Stimulating Solution is totally natural, as such will be more effective for you if you have a proper diet and stay away from these chemicals.

General Health

Your metabolism produces energy, which is used during sex. I am not referring to crazy competitive fucking. Increased arousal and the resulting physiologic changes such as increased blood pressure and increased breathing rate can be surprisingly tiring. Lethargy and energy depletion can cause a faster than normal climax sensitivity.

As a result, if you are not healthy enough, you might be prone to cumming against your will. Some obese men are also likely to cum quickly. Your choice of diet can be more tiring than nourishing.

Experts suggest that a proper diet provides nourishment and can determine sexual health. The pathways involved in sex can be stimulated by moderate exercise. If you are trying to repair one cylinder of a V8 engine, it might never function effectively if the others are weak.

Masturbation Habits

Can you recall being a teenager and frantically rushing to cum before you are discovered by anyone, worst-case scenario, your mom? According to some experts, constantly hurrying to finish could be responsible for premature ejaculation by conditioning you to climax very fast. Even if this behavior does not always cause premature ejaculation, it may aggravate or potentiate it. Research has discovered that there are similarities in the way men masturbate, regardless of whether they have premature ejaculation or not. We generally use a similar intensity and degree of physical stimulation.

The variation is in using visual stimulation such as pornography, for instance. Some studies have discovered that the inclusion of visual stimulation to physical stimulation results in a fall in control of ejaculation, so the likelihood of premature ejaculation becomes higher. Therefore, premature ejaculation is likely to happen when you have a mixture of physical (reflexive) stimulation and mental (visual or psychogenic) stimulation.

This is a significant discovery because the treatment techniques of premature ejaculation are centered on a type of meditation-based awareness practiced while masturbating. This might be effective when it is just you and your penis involved, but the majority of guys masturbate using pornography or other visual stimulation. Including that type of psychogenic stimulation to the combination and awareness training might be ineffective. The chances that this would be successful with a partner are even lower.

Increased Sensitivity of the Penis

There is a probability that there is an increased sensitivity of the penis of men with premature ejaculation and this explains why they ejaculate too soon. This hypothesis is supported by some research compared them to guys that do not have premature ejaculations. Men with chronic premature ejaculation have been discovered to have an increased sensitivity of the penis. Sprays, creams, and other chemicals used to reduce sensations in the penis have been moderately effective.

Additionally, there is proof that suggests the opposite, that there is reduced penis sensitivity of guys with premature ejaculation. Recent research published in the Journal of Sexual Medicine studied 83 men; of which about 50% of them had premature ejaculation while the rest did not have any ejaculatory problems. The scientist's utilized equipment that applied cold, vibratory, and hot sensations to the penises of the men to measure the sensitivity.

After five tests, it was discovered that men with premature ejaculation seemed to have reduced sensitivity in their penises. This does not imply that the numbing chemicals would be ineffective for these men; it just suggests that increased sensitivity of the penis does not necessarily cause premature ejaculation.

Psychological Blocks

Performance, especially sexual performance, is determined by the mental state. I am going with the optimistic ideology whereby using this book you can effectively retrain your mind. However, it is important to note that a deep mental issue can impede your progress. A percentage of men occasionally cum too quickly due to untreated psychological problems.

Throughout history, premature ejaculation was regarded as an emotional problem deeply rooted in psychological issues such as guilt, the fear of failure, rejection, anxiety about under-performing, depression, personal and relationship problems and stress (even regarding other unconnected issues). Though men with chronic premature ejaculation might actually experience these problems, they are tempted to manage their premature ejaculation but are not directly responsible. A few therapies that could be helpful in treating these negative energies are:

- Tantric Sexual Healing

- Personal Counseling

- Relationship Counseling

- Reduction of Traumatic Incident

If you are not noticing any improvements after all these or you are finding it difficult to follow the program, consider seeing a sex therapist or any other specialist.

Relationship Distress

Premature ejaculation may be caused by complex interpersonal issues. Relationship distress premature ejaculation is caused by interpersonal issues, such as poor communication, extreme discomfort or fear of sex, fear of relationship success, intense sensitivity to your partner, hurtful disagreements, unsettled emotional conflicts, or lack of trust due to infidelity.

In a nutshell, general relationship inadequacies antagonize the common emotional acceptance that is necessary for sexual health. Even if premature ejaculation is due to a different reason outside relationship distress, it can significantly destroy your relationship nonetheless. Relationship distress PE is restricted to sex with that partner and is usually acquired.

Although, there is no general pattern among couples experiencing premature ejaculation, there are numerous common patterns.

- The man is extremely sensitive to his partner and is afraid of failing and performing below her expectations, so he constantly blames himself and is remorseful.

- The woman might be direct and quarrelsome or timid and submissive.

- The man is selfish and detached from his partner's needs. He might make excuses for his problems as a regular biological response, while she might feel emotionally neglected and unwanted and becomes antagonistic.

- The couple suffers from unsettled emotional conflicts

in addition to engaging in criticism, blaming, and neglect.

- They might find it difficult to balance independence with couple unity, conflict-solving deadlock, and lack of empathy. One partner might feel neglected by the other and become aggressive or unbothered.

As you can see, premature ejaculation might be a mutual and interactive issue that is related to a relationship problem rather than the actual act of sex. Sexual dysfunction such as premature ejaculation could be an alternate issue, creating a focus for the anxiety and discontent issues of the couple, thereby creating the illusion that other aspects of the relationship are intact. It may feel like sex is the only issue, but this usually not true.

Inexperience

A common misconception is that premature ejaculation is limited to young men. Some people have put forward a hypothesis that men with premature ejaculation are not very experienced sexually, and are unaware of their arousal; this is not true at all. Actually, research has discovered that men with premature ejaculation use the same degree of stimulation during masturbation as men without premature ejaculation. There is no actual difference in self-awareness and skill between men with mature ejaculation and those without.

Premature ejaculation is not caused by sexual ignorance, but it could explain the reason for a lack of absolute control over the time taken to orgasm. Ejaculation mastery develops with age and experience. You become better as you grow older.

Change in a Sexual Partner

Consciously, or otherwise, sexual partners have some form of expectations from men, whether they vocalize it or the man interprets it mentally. Still, it is present. Under normal conditions, especially in exclusive sexual relationships, there is a reduction in the level of subtle expectation with consistent sex with the same partner. This creates a sense of intimacy, comfort, and self-confidence. Changing partners might result in new feelings of anxiety, fear, pressure, and intimidation, which might result in premature ejaculation.

In the same way, the opposite is true. That is, as we have seen before, if you are living in a toxic relationship, the mental pressure and stress regarding expectations could negatively affect the Cum.
In extreme cases, it has been proven that men trapped in harmful relationships, have never suffered from PE again when changing partners.

Malconditioning

A young man might be inhibited from exploring his sexual abilities by his rigorous and restrained upbringing. Additionally, sexual trauma, e.g., being discovered during masturbation, and imbibing wrong habits e.g., masturbating very fast to prevent being caught, may condition unhealthy reactions to sexual stimulation.

Medical Causes

Though medical conditions account for only a few cases of PE, such conditions must not be treated lightly in order to manage PE cases. Such medical issues include injuries to the nervous system, side effects from medications, trauma, physical injuries, post-surgical effects, or effects of substance abuse.

Physical Injury PE

Physical injury (temporary or permanent) accounts for some of the cases of PE. For instance, direct or indirect injury to the testes could affect the ejaculatory system. Also, injury to the nerves that connect the genitals to the nervous system could affect the conduction of impulses to and from the genitals thereby compromising sensation/stimulation and ejaculation.

Drug Side-Effect PE

The use of or withdrawal from certain pharmaceutical agents could lead to PE. Such conditions are acquired. Some examples include the use of nonprescription cold medicines such as pseudoephedrine (Sudafed) and withdrawal from opiates or tranquilizers.

Chapter 3:

Recognizing Premature Ejaculation

It is all too common to find many individuals worry unnecessarily due to self-diagnosis. Before you conclude that you have PE, it is imperative to carry out a performance test and seek your partner's opinion in order to prevent unnecessary negative feelings. Also, check some of the signs of PE listed below:

- Failure to know when you're about to ejaculate

- Early ejaculation or orgasm within 1-2 minutes of masturbation or penetration

- Inability to delay ejaculation during masturbation or sex

- Persistent dissatisfaction of yourself or partner dissatisfaction after sex

How Does Premature Ejaculation Affect You?

Generally, persistent and chronic PE poses three major challenges:

- It affects how long a person will last before orgasm.

- It determines whether or not an individual can delay ejaculation.

- It affects the personality of the individual negatively.

Let's analyze these challenges one at a time.

You don't last long

Most men assume that sex does last for hours based on what they see in movies or what they hear from their boastful colleagues in the locker room. On Average, most men last for 2-5 minutes before ejaculation but men with PE last for less than one minute.

There is scientific evidence to back this fact up. Scientists developed a device known as the Intravaginal Ejaculatory Latency Time (IELT), which can be used to estimate how long a man lasts during intercourse before ejaculation. Though various researchers gave different times, on average, men with PE usually lasted between 15-60 seconds.

I have seen various cases of PE, and some are so serious that they reach climax or orgasm even before penetration, cumming after mere heavy petting or direct manual stimulation. As a result of this, they can't explore the full pleasure of their sexual potential. In the end, they leave their mate dissatisfied and find it hard to explain why they can't accept any form of sexual stimulation from their partner.

You can't hold back

Men with PE can't hold back from ejaculating no matter how hard they try, and the "think about baseball" trick doesn't work for them. There's no universal ejaculating threshold (the amount of stimulation required before ejaculation) for all men where ejaculation is inevitable. But for men with PE, the threshold is notably quite low, and some people orgasm immediately after penetration.

On the other hand, women have no business with ejaculatory inevitability and can lose an orgasm at the point when it's happening. Most women don't understand the concept of ejaculatory threshold and ejaculatory inevitability, thus why they always want to turn their partner on.

Telling a man with PE to wait until he's ready to orgasm is one of the worst things a woman can say, as the stress of waiting will likely increase the rate of ejaculatory inevitability. Each woman differs from the other and her ability to orgasm also differs, so you can't just assume you have PE because you couldn't get your partner to orgasm before you orgasm.

Some women orgasm within a short time while others can't orgasm through sexual intercourse because it takes a longer time to reach that threshold. But generally, men with PE won't hold up long enough to satisfy their partner via vaginal intercourse and this is the reason why most of the men with PE constantly worry about their sexual failure.

PE affects your life.

Not being able to hold back or last long makes a man with PE lose his sexual confidence, and such feelings can bring about a lot of negative emotions in these men. They might feel insecure, frustrated, embarrassed, worried and angry with themselves.

Most of the men with PE are worried about what their partner will think of them, especially partners who don't understand the concept of PE. These men might fear they will be tagged as sexually selfish or just plain lazy. The truth is that men with PE are usually sensitive lovers; they just lack the ability to put that positive energy into action and instead consciously try to hold back for too long taking the pleasure out of sex altogether. In the end, most men with PE start avoiding relationships, sexual situations, and even women in general.

From my experience, most women who are unaware of the condition of their partner usually complain about how distant and depressed their partner is and how he avoids sex. Sadly, this is not limited to affecting the relationship with just that partner. It also affects the relationship between the man affected with PE and his wider friendship circle. Once his friends start talking about their own sexual escapades, such men with PE feel withdrawn because they see themselves as being left out or less of a man.

Premature ejaculation can make a man feel this lonely because he feels no one can understand him even if he tries to talk about it. He might feel sexually incapacitated, immature and out of control.

Developing Realistic Sexual Expectations

In order to learn ejaculatory control, first, you need to fill your mind with realistic expectations rather than expecting more from your body than it is biologically and functionally designed to do. In this section, we will examine your personal expectations when it comes to sex.

Exercise: Assessing Your Expectations During Sex

What are your expectations when it comes to your sexual life? Are those expectations the same as what other couples expect? Are they positive, realistic expectations? If yes, what are they? Below are some known facts about couple sexuality and expectations.

Frequency

This has to do with how often you have sex. What are some factors that can influence the frequency? Such factors include:

- The quality of your relationship

- Your body's sexual urge

- The balance between work and leisure time

- The agreements between you and your partner

But what does it mean if you're having more or less sex than you and your mate expect?

On average, married couples have sex about four times a week and a minimum of once a week. Despite popular belief, married couples that live together are actually both more sexually active and satisfied than unmarried couples living together or those that are dating. According to the research conducted by Michael *et al.* (1994), married couples in their 20s have sex about 2-3 times a week while those in their 50s have sex at least once a week. The research revealed that couples that have sex less than twice a month are more likely to find it difficult to master and maintain ejaculatory control. If you have sex frequently, you'll develop a sort of sexual rhythm that will help you have better control over your ejaculation.

Length

One of the most controversial questions about sex is: How long should sexual intercourse last? One, two, five or 30 minutes? Other related questions include: What is the link between the quality of sex and the duration? And what does the length of sex mean for you?

Typically, an average sexual escapade should last between 15-45 minutes out of which 2-7 minutes will involve the actual penetration of intercourse (Leiblum and Rosen, 1989). However, a sexual encounter could vary between a two-minute quickie to a deep, erotic, sensual and intimate, two-hour escapade. The act of lovemaking involves both nonverbal and verbal communication, foreplay, intercourse, pleasuring, and after play. One shocking lie that the media often portrays is about how men can last for several minutes to hours, but the truth is that most men don't last for more than 10 minutes of thrusting after which the swagger drops. Such facts and figures are shocking for most men and women.

In my opinion, forget the time, forget the focus of penetration. Are you excited? Then play with her, with her and your body. Personally, I enjoy arousing my woman with kisses, caresses and other types of erotic activities even for an entire hour. I'm getting closer and closer to her intimate area, but without going in. Then I constantly change position, from the bed we go to stand up, then maybe we dance naked and attached with the music chosen for that moment. Then I change again; for me it's almost an exercise where I have to let my imagination run wild. Everyone knows more or less how to penetrate a female, but how many know how to roam the world around her. I call myself an explorer, it's more fun. They appreciate it. Sometimes, with this mentality, with this kind of foreplay, the woman can get so excited that at the moment of penetration, it only takes one, and I repeat, only one push, which have already reached orgasm.

Arousal

Ask yourself, what condition(s) induce(s) an erection in you as male? When do you find it more difficult to be turned on? What does it mean when you find it difficult to get an erection? What does it mean if your erection dwindles before and/or during sex?

It might interest you to know that occasionally arousal failure can occur in the form of failed erection, and this can even happen in the middle of intercourse. Instead of panicking, why not continue with erotic but nonintercourse sex until either one or both of you orgasm.

Get out of your head that sex or making love is just penetration. Our body is full of nerve endings and stimulation points. Explore the potential of your body and that of your body. Develop and exercise your imagination. Don't sadly limit yourself to penetration alone to express your passion for her. The possibilities are so wide that they border on infinity. Try to think of this example, in geometry it is established that a line between point A and point B is formed by "infinite number of points".

Now you can imagine how the possible combinations existing between two human bodies included in bed can be much more than multiple. It would not be enough for us to discover them all in one lifetime.

As far as I'm concerned, I believe that the Kamasutra (with all due respect) represents only one small index of initiation into sex.

I repeat: TWO BODIES AND INFINITE POSSIBILITY OF GAME.

Ejaculatory Control

What are your expectations regarding ejaculatory control and how realistic are they? How do you determine this? If you ejaculate fast, what does it mean? How much control are you expected to have over ejaculation? Who is expected to time ejaculation?

What about PE, how do you know when you're cured? What does it mean to have a 'reasonable' level of control over when to be orgasmic? What is a reasonable and realistic expectation about orgasms for women? These are all questions you might ask about ejaculatory control.

One simple way forward is to ensure that you focus on feeling pleasure during intercourse. As long as both you and your partner are satisfied with sexual pleasures, ejaculatory control should be the least of your worries.

Another clue to answering these questions is to ensure that intercourse is an interactive and mutual experience. Most men are able to identify the point of ejaculatory inevitability, and they've been able to learn how to slow down and control ejaculation both with oral and manual stimulation. To properly manage this condition, it requires both interaction and cooperation from both partners.

Satisfaction

What do you expect before you can be emotionally and sexually satisfied? Is ejaculation compulsory? Must every sexual intercourse be equally satisfying? Why do you feel distressed over a poor sexual experience? What do you think about just pleasing your partner (mercy sex)?

Research has shown that even among sexually active, satisfied married couples, half (or fewer) of them are equally satisfied. Any couple that enjoys quality sex in which both partners are satisfied should count themselves lucky. In about 20-25% of marriages, only one couple gets satisfied (usually the man) and another 20-25% of sexual experiences are good enough but not extraordinary.

It is also important to understand that only about five to 15% of sexual experiences are dysfunctional, mediocre, or dissatisfying. Keep in mind that this is the truth for satisfied and well-functioning couples.

Don't get me wrong. I'm not saying that sometimes you have to settle for it. What I want to express is that many times we men care much more about what we should.
This prevents us from flowing into what corresponds to the beautiful energy of sex, passion and Kundalini. I just want you to try to push yourself beyond the normal paradigms in which we grew up. The benefits we can derive from a good and conscious sexual energy can completely change our lives, for the better of course.

Unfortunately, in this consumer society, there are those who do not want you to be aware. Our economic system needs compulsive consumers, early ejaculators of consumption. Learn to know and control your mind, otherwise someone else will do it for you.

Chapter 4:

Enjoying Sex and Preventing Relapse

Learning ejaculatory control requires effort, time, energy, and cooperation and you can't afford to relapse. Assuming that one bout of PE relapse is impossible would amount to deceiving oneself. Occasionally pushing couples to resort to the blame and counter-blame cycle. Therefore, you should have positive and realistic expectations while also accepting the ideology that orgasm and arousal are inherently variable.

Occasionally, you might experience bouts of rapid ejaculation (one every 10 times, once in a month, or once each year). Such occurrences are totally normal and there is no need to panic. In fact, such things are part of some couple's sexual journey. The best way to go about this is to accept such occasional episodes as normal, but don't allow them to become a norm (relapse).

In the course of this chapter, you will learn how to develop and implement a personal and specific relapse prevention strategy. It is imperative for you to handle a PE situation when it occurs rather than simply assume that it will never happen again. Don't worry we will discuss the important measures needed to prevent a relapse.

The Basis of Relapse Prevention

With PE, you need to acquire the knowledge of how to prevent relapse. You've already learned about the various factors that contribute to PE; how couples can build a sexual style that integrates intimacy with team models of change; and how to have realistic expectations of ejaculatory control. With all these resources at your disposal, we will now address how to prevent relapse using cognitive, behavioral, and emotional approaches.

The Cognitive Foundation of Relapse Prevention

Accepting the fact that you will rapidly ejaculate occasionally is the best cognitive strategy to prevent relapse. When you view such experiences as part of a normal variation, other than a sign of performance or anticipatory anxiety, such positive thinking will help you and your partner to view such variations as a moment in time rather than a relapse. With that in mind, you will be able to cognitively handle subsequent encounter(s) positively, feeling more relaxed while you engage in self-entrancement arousal and enjoy the pleasurable buildup of the stimulation. With this in mind you can then apply some of the strategies with intention and clear headedly, such as the start-stop or slow-down pacing to see your awareness of the rate of intercourse thrusting.

An important method for preventing relapse is to redirect your focus from performance-oriented sex towards the active involvement in the entire process of lovemaking and the display of affection during and after play. Sexual intercourse is a continuation of pleasure, intimacy, and eroticism. It is not a pass-fail test but an extension of the pleasuring process. Keep in mind that the duration of intercourse varies based on your desires. With the new set of skills you're acquiring, you will be able to maintain a reasonable level of control over when you ejaculate. Have it at the back of your mind that you and your partner are involved in the process and you're not just performing a show for her.

Rather than view your partner as a demanding master whom you must please, why not view her as an intimate friend whose arousal and pleasures are needed to feed yours and vice versa? To enjoy satisfying intercourse, both of you don't need to orgasm at the same time, in a certain sequence, all you need is for you to enjoy each other's arousal.

Our idea of a good-enough sexual relationship and good-enough ejaculatory control is to enjoy pleasurable sex and not to obtain a perfect sexual experience every time. This realistic cognitive thinking will enable you to gain better control over a relapse.

The Behavioral Basis of Relapse Prevention

Ensuring your confidence and comfort is the most important behavioral approach for the prevention of relapses coupled with arousal spacing and the stop-start techniques. You'll learn these skills while discussing the systematic ejaculatory control exercises. But the major challenge is how to apply what you'll learn during a spontaneous bout of intercourse in order to enjoy and maintain good-enough ejaculatory control. It is imperative to apply this technique in your sex life. If you and your partner have taken a break from your sexual rhythm, you can decide to implement this skill once you resume sexual activities. In the meantime, do it in a more structured manner.

Your aim should be to enjoy a form of a sexual encounter in which you enjoy pleasurable and relaxing foreplay of anything from touching to erotic arousal. Give and receive pleasures then transition into the actual sexual intercourse while monitoring your pelvic muscles (PM) until you both climax with orgasmic satisfaction emotionally, relationally, and physically.

To properly manage PE and gain ejaculatory control, there is a need for regular rhythmic sexual experiences. Both partners need to be involved and continually aware, or else, you might risk regression to PE.

The Emotional Basis of Relapse Prevention

There's a strong link between what you feel for each other and your sexual life. You need to value and strengthen your bond of friendship and your interpersonal relationship if you wish to have a healthy sexual life. Another important area involves setting aside time for some quality couple talk which will help deepen your bond of intimacy. With the right amount of commitment, you can both enjoy a flexible emotional intimacy, filled with eroticism and pleasure.

Basic Concepts Necessary for Ejaculatory Control

Even as you work as a team to maintain ejaculatory control and improve your sexual style as a couple, you still need to recall the key concepts you learned earlier. Going through your record, which concepts proved to be the most challenging one for you to learn and master? Such concepts require your utmost attention and you need to rehearse it more to prevent a relapse.

Many young males start as rapid ejaculators making PE the major sexuality issue in males. In addition, 30% of adult males experience PE.

Therefore, having a realistic expectation cannot be overemphasized. Base your expectations on your physical abilities and the biological makeup of your body.

The do-it-yourself techniques as a form of arousal control will not help you gain ejaculatory control, but rather interfere with the process of arousal leading to possible erectile dysfunction.

The best approach for ejaculatory control is sometimes counterintuitive. Your goal shouldn't be to decrease pleasure; rather, you want to boost your pleasure, comfort, and awareness.

One vital skill you need to master while trying to gain ejaculatory control is to find a balance between sensual self-entrancement, physical relaxation during intercourse, and partner interaction arousal.

To fully gain ejaculatory control, you need to know the point of ejaculatory inevitability, and then maintain a high level of awareness during arousal.

That said, having ejaculatory control in the middle of partner sex can be very complicated and tasking.

The aim of ejaculatory control is to boost pleasure and eroticism between the both of you. It is not to merely ensure your partner has a multiple orgasm during lovemaking, because at least one out of every four women respond to orgasms in the same manner as men (just one orgasm during lovemaking).

There are three time-tested and effective behavioral tools that can help improve ejaculatory control. They include:

- Pelvic muscle relaxation

- The stop-start technique

- The intercourse acclimation technique

Ejaculatory control can't be learned and mastered immediately, it is a gradual learning process and so continual practice and feedback is necessary.

Try as much as possible to relax your pelvic muscle as much as you can once you initiate lovemaking, so your body can have enough levels of ejaculatory control.

In the beginning when you start learning ejaculatory control, let the woman take the top position and allow enough time to adapt to the learning process. Other sexual positions are more tasking. Also, you could try the circular or longer, slower method of thrusting. Don't forget to take turns in doing the thrusting. During short and rapid thrusting with the man-on-top position, ejaculatory control is very difficult.

The sensations of orgasm commence from the point of ejaculatory inevitability. This is the point of no return and it is totally out of your control, but you *can* determine how you react at this point. Try as much as possible to enjoy the pleasures of the moment rather than being unnecessarily angry with yourself for PE.

The physical, emotional, and sexual satisfaction of your partner is equally important. Hence, you can pleasure her to arousal until she attains orgasm by orally or manually rubbing sensitive areas or by using vibrator stimulation. Some women prefer such acts after ejaculation (but most prefer it before sex).

If PE is caused by a neurological condition, you can decide to use medications as an additional resource while you still practice ejaculatory control exercises. Once you notice that you're gaining control, you can gradually stop taking the medications. Always discuss these transitions with your doctor first.

I am absolutely against the use of drugs but in extreme cases, extreme remedies!

Remember, sexuality is not only about performing perfectly but also involves giving and receiving pleasure. So try to enjoy the entire lovemaking experience: pleasure, intimacy, arousal, eroticism, intercourse, and after play, laughing, joking and even pausing to hydrate or catch your breath.

Relapse Prevention Strategies

To overcome relapse, both partners need to be committed by devoting their time and energy to ensure they enjoy high-grade intimacy. This requires that they maintain a regular rhythm of playful, passionate, sensual, sexual bonds—three times a week or at the very least, once in ten days—rather than going back to the intercourse-or-nothing style. To be clear, healthy sexuality goes beyond frequency, because there are other contributing factors that need to be attended to such as noting your physical health and habits (as mentioned before: eating healthy, not smoking, regular exercise, moderate to no drinking, and a healthy sleep pattern). Also, you might need to go for regular checkups at the local health center to ensure that an infection or any side effects from medication do not affect your sexuality. Now, let us look at ten specific relapse prevention approaches that could be of help to you.

Hold regular couple meetings

Working as a close team is very important if you want to have a healthy, intimate relationship. Having regular times (for instance, the last day of every month) to discuss your sexuality as a couple will help you learn ejaculatory control much faster and improve the level of communication as a couple.

Hold an official follow-up meeting

Holding regular meetings every six months to monitor your progress as a couple or with a therapist will help both of you to remain accountable and committed to having good-quality, erotic, and enjoyable sex. It will also help prevent a relapse because both of you will be more cautious not to slip back into unhealthy sexual feelings, behaviors, and attitudes. The worst mistake a couple can ever make is to treat PE and intimacy flippantly.

Have special pleasuring moments

Carving out time for a pleasuring session without orgasm enhances communication, playfulness, and sensuality. Such moments allow couples to enjoy pure sensuality. You will be able to try out new styles in the meantime, such as the use of body lotions, alternative pleasuring positions, or new settings. This will help you to focus on flexibility and pleasuring rather than perfection. Nurturing and maintaining sensuality and pleasuring helps to prevent relapse not only for PE but also for other sexual challenges.

Humbly accept your lapses as mere tests

Change doesn't happen instantly. As in any change process, there are times when lapses will occur, so it is important to view such lapses as a test and not a sign of failure.

To achieve a reasonable level of success, you need to be challenged. Whenever your new skill is put to the test and you handle it well, it will help boost your confidence and you will be better prepared to handle subsequent difficulties. Your progress becomes more visible and your goal more achievable. You can then say with confidence that you have mastered the skills of sexual intimacy and cooperation.

Even after learning and mastering how to control PE, most

couples will likely be tested at least twice. The most common test is a relapse experience of PE, which could be as severe as the bad old days. At such moments, various questions could come to your mind, such as: Are we back to where we started? Why did the method fail? Will I ever overcome PE?

When you're tested like this, the most important thing is for you to endure together. You can do this by sharing physical feelings and emotions, always being understanding as well as applying all the other skills you'll learn from this book. Instead of feeling angry, frustrated, or disappointed, why not keep the fire going by touching, pleasuring, and taking time to relax your bodies. You can also focus on relaxing your PM before you initiate intercourse, making love more slowly, allowing more time for vaginal acclimation, or using circular intercourse motions. You should also always discuss the sexual events after the fact. Maybe even laugh off the experience before you prepare for the next encounter (likely within the next three days when you have regained your energy) of slow, sensual, and erotic lovemaking.

Hold reasonable expectations

By now, we hope your idea of movie-quality erections and sex that lasts for hours have faded away. Sex serves several purposes besides pleasure. Sex can be used to relieve stress, settle a dispute, show affection or appreciation, bridge the gap caused by emotional distance, or to share intimacy even if one partner enjoys sex more than the other.

Make plans for intimate couple time

Even after years of marriage, couples still need to set aside quality time for each other. This time needs to be exclusively the couple and with no distractions from the children or the outside world. You need some quality time to groom your relationship. Most couples often report that they enjoy quality sex when they go on vacation. Similar times could be spent taking a walk, going out for dinner, or discussing intimate matters.

It is essential for a couple, not to give up these moments of intimacy. They must never be left on the sidelines of a habitual life full of superficial problems. Giving oneself sacred moments of intimacy in a constant way, almost as if it were a ritual, is the secret for the healing of conflicts and possible misunderstandings. These moments allow the marriage to continue to vibrate at the same frequency.

Allow time to pass to develop your couple sexual style

When it comes to sexuality, there is no hard and fast rule as to how to initiate sex, create erotic scenes and styles, have intercourse, or engage in after play. This gives a chance for flexibility and change in your own time and helps prevent relapse.

There are no sexual experiences outside the world, we are all human beings, with our weaknesses and our merits. Although sometimes certain situations in which you dive, may seem to you to the limit of the unlikely, think that you are not the first and you will not even be the last.

Quality sex ranges from manageable to great

Preparing for negative sexual experiences or disappointments will help you cope with relapse. Not all sexual experiences are out of this world. Also, the way you respond to any disappointing situations matters most. The ability to properly manage and not overreact under such circumstances will help you prevent relapse.

Enjoy sensual, erotic touching

Intimacy involves sexuality but goes beyond just sexual intercourse. You and your partner need different erotic and intimate ways to bond and maintain the bond. Such erotic bonds include affectionate touching, non-orgasmic pleasuring, sensual stimulation, and lovemaking. These are great to use and enjoy as you work on your new techniques for PE control.

Continue expanding your sexual potential

Maintaining an erotic relationship and sexual flexibility is important if you want to prevent a relapse. Great sex must be able to satisfy a wide range of needs, feelings, and help you gain and maintain ejaculatory control. Couples that enjoy playful intimacy such as semi-clothed cuddling, massages, bathing together, holding hands, and naked sensual touches have a more flexible sexual repertoire. Mix it up. Couples that engage in quickies, prolonged and erotic foreplays, planned *and* spontaneous sexual intercourse are reported to enjoy a robust sexual relationship.

Have you ever tried to focus on your own breath and her breath? Controlling your breathing, bringing it to a slow and deep rhythm in sync with your partner is one of the most beautiful ways in my opinion, to establish a bond and get down together within your bodies.

Bringing attention to breathing is an important key to distract yourself from those that are projections of the mind and live the present moment.

Chapter 5:

Communication is Key

Communication is vital in all areas of our lives. To keep a healthy and satisfying sexual relationship, communication is just as essential between the parties involved. However, most problems in relationships are a result of the man's wounded ego from his failure to sexually satisfy his partner and his subsequent inability to talk about the problem.

A man would rather remain quiet than discuss his sexual problems such as early ejaculation to anyone, including his partner. This is because of the general notion that a man should be able to control his sexual stimulation or arousal. Therefore, any man who is not in control of himself is supposedly not man enough. This notion has caused a lot of men to feel ashamed to talk to someone about their sexual inabilities, causing more harm than cure.

Turning a blind eye or refusing to acknowledge a problem does not solve the problem, it worsens the situation. In the case of sexual problems, refusing to acknowledge these problems could make the situation more irritating and create emotional stress, misunderstandings, hurt feelings, and anger. Talking to your partner, and in some cases, a doctor could help not just you but others who are suffering from the same problem. Being able to open to someone brings more advantages than disadvantages.

Sex can be good sometimes and other times, sex can be bad. Sex can be quick, and sex can be slow. It all depends on individual preferences. Sex is not a topic to be worried over as much as some people do. This section emphasizes communication as a way to enjoy your relationship beyond sex.

Communication With Your Spouse

Research has shown that couples that discuss their sexual problems, especially that of the male, have a better chance of handling the situation and coming out stronger. As a couple, the problem of one partner is the problem of the other. So, the best way to deal with it is as a couple. Men who tell their partners about their sexual dysfunction usually realize that their partners are willing to help and are also interested in improving their sexual life. This alone encourages the man and makes it simpler for the couple to find solutions to the problem.

The hardest discussion a man can have with his partner is one involving his sexual inabilities. Telling your partner that you are having premature ejaculation could be the hardest thing you've ever done. Since your partner has already noticed this problem, in most cases, deciding to talk about it as a couple can feel even more shameful. Most men feel it is embarrassing to acknowledge that they cannot satisfy their partners in bed, but the best thing is to let them know. This way, you both understand yourselves and work towards finding solutions. Opening up to your partner not only relieves you of your worries but it will also provide you with support in looking for a way out.

Tips for Talking With Your Partner

- Do not hide your feelings from your partner. Be open; make sure your partner knows how you feel.

- When talking to your partner about your sexual

problems, make sure you do not cast blame; instead, discuss how to solve the issue, what you both want and your goals as a couple so you can work towards achieving them.

- While you and your partner are still searching for a cure, emphasize that you can try out other sexual practices to gain sexual satisfaction in the meantime.

- You should make clear you priority in achieving a healthy sexual life. You can show your commitment to the cause by discussing seeking medical attention and advice.

Communicate to Cut Down Stress

There are many reasons for premature ejaculation but for some men, stress is one of the major causes. However, the simplest therapy for reducing stress is talking to someone you can trust about the problems you are worrying over. This will not just relieve you of your current worries, it could also help in solving other problems simultaneously.

Obviously, try to choose the right person. Someone who aims at your interests and not his own. A person who can enhance your perception of reality. Someone who is ready to listen, understand and help you with advice based on experience and not on "hearsay".

Communicating Based on Differences

Communication between the male sex female sexes can be difficult because these two can sometimes seem so different. It can feel like you are two different species, making communication between you and your woman difficult. Not being able to communicate effectively is one of the main reasons why most relationships hit the rocks or crash.

However, there are some things you can do as a man to make communication with your partner a whole lot easier despite your differences. These things are quite easy, and they will help you to enjoy your relationship more.

On top of acknowledging your problems delaying ejaculation, you also must accept that your partner does not go through the same things you do. She reacts differently to things. You must accept that these differences will always be there. Women tend to curl up and become cold emotionally if they feel their emotions are taken for granted or that their partners are not paying attention to their feelings or what they have to say. Problems like these could lead to frustration in the relationship. It could also result in the refusal to indulge in any sexual act, which is essential in most relationships. You can only break this chain with communication and respect of your differences.

The simplest solution to this problem is paying attention to your woman. Listen to whatever she has to say, whether it makes sense or not. Give her your full attention. Sometimes a woman starts up a conversation that might not be very relevant at the time; it could be a story, what is bothering her, or her fears or concerns. All she wants is to have your attention. Show her that you are interested in whatever she has to say. Women crave an emotional connection with their partner and one way to achieve this is by communication.

Effective communication is an essential part of any good relationship. Once the communication aspect of your relationship is healthy, then all other aspects can be worked out. Communication is the bedrock of any relationship. Feelings can be nurtured when communication is in place and feelings can wear off once communication is out of the picture. Other factors like stress and worries, can make partners feel distant from each other and the only way to reduce this stress is by opening up to each other and talking about your similarities as well as your differences.

Be sincere enough to open to your partner about your fears, concerns, and desires too. This way, both of you will be able to manage the situation and understand yourselves and each other better.

In sexual relationships, if the problems noticed or experienced during an intimate session are not discussed openly between the two parties, it could result in emotional tension, which could eventually lead to break up. If you are both open you can try to improve your sexual relationship. Once communicating and committed to improving your relationship, you and your sexual partner can try the following tips.

How to Help a Woman Relax

Stress from work and other commitments, both internal and external can throw a woman into a state of unrest. This will, in turn, drive her attention away from any intimate or sexual act. So, in order to get through to your partner, you have to help reduce her stress and help her to relax.

Try some of the following to relax your partner:

- A good massage on her neck or back

- A sensual foot massage

- A warm bath with her

- Caressing her hair while she is listening to her favorite song

It is important to state here that these measures are different for different women. What this means is, what works for your friend's partner might not work for yours. Communication comes into play yet again. Talk with her and most importantly *listen* to her to find out ways you can help her relax.

A massage or bath will begin to relax the body. But in order for a woman's body to be completely at rest, her mind must be relaxed too. Both mind and body must be at ease to help her become sexually excited. The mind consists of the five senses: smell, hearing, touch, taste, and sight. Understanding the part each of these senses plays can help you and your partner reach ultimate relaxation.

The Five Senses

In this section, I will discuss the roles each sense plays in relaxing a woman.

Sight

Women are attracted to looks and physical appearances. But most importantly, women pay attention to the surrounding environment. They take note of the state of your home, whether it is tidy, or it looks like a pig's pen. They tend to feel more comfortable and relaxed in a clean home, especially the bedroom where sexual acts can take place. Keeping your house clean is essential if you want your partner to feel at home. It sounds simple enough, but can make a world of difference. Change the dirty bed sheets, arrange your wardrobe, and pick up any underwear or clothing littering your floor. Show her that you can take care of yourself and your home and she will trust you can take care of her too.

Hearing

Simple sounds can relax and arouse a woman. Sounds like soft, love-filled music in the background or a sweet compliment whispered in her ears can work wonders to relax your partner and ultimately get her into the mood.

Taste

Taste should not be ignored. Taste buds can be your ticket to a sexually excited woman. Try out new foods and snacks like chocolates, cheese, berries, and assorted wines. This can ignite her senses and help set up a romantic environment, eventually leading to a wonderful sexual experience.

Smell

In seducing a woman, the sense of smell plays a very vital role. Most women appreciate perfume gifts. But, a man's scent can excite a woman too. It has a way of putting her in the mood. Once you smell delicious, add some sweet smelling candles to the environment to stir up sexual feelings and romance even more.

Touch

Once you've relaxed her other senses, then you can start with touch. Touching, we already know, can relax her body. But don't dive right into the sensitive spots. You can start by holding her hands to clear her doubts and gain trust. Listen to her body language and movements. Women are very sensitive to touch and they have different ways of showing it. She might begin to breath quickly or deeply. Use this and verbal communication to know when to move on to other areas. Her body and her words will tell you where she wants and how she wants it.

How to Relax Her Body

We already know that the mind and body affect each other in achieving relaxation. You have learned a few tricks to relax the body and diverse ways you can relax her mind. Let's look at a few more ways to incorporate touch into relaxing your partner's body.

The right kind of touch can show your partner there is nowhere else in the world you'd rather be than with her. Kissing, touching, and authentic eye contact can make her feel like the only one, which helps her to relax her mind leading to a more relaxed body. But these simple acts can do more than help her relax. Showing that you love and want them can be enough to arouse a woman sexually.

Planned sexual acts are not always the best. Make a point to kiss your partner when she least expects, learn to steal kisses from her when she's talking, working, or just not expecting it. Hold her hands while kissing her or gently caress her face. It sounds simple, but all these little actions will help to build up sexual desire and excitement.

Foreplay is a sexual act meant to relax a woman's body and prepare her for sex. When doing this, you must be careful to touch all parts of her body including her stomach, waist, and feet. Leave no part untouched (or unkissed). The following tips will help you focus your touch depending on the area.

Shoulders and neck

These two parts can be very sensitive to touch. If touched skillfully, you can easily relax and arouse your woman. Take time to caress your woman's shoulders and neck with your fingers *and* your tongue. And don't forget the kisses!

Ears

Ears are another extremely sensitive place to remember. Take time to touch her ears with the tip of your fingers and your tongue. Play with her ear lobes as well, as the lower part of the ear is the most sensitive. If she has long hair, pick up the hair softly and gently kiss her ears, moving down to her neck and shoulders. In addition to kissing and touching, simply breathing can do the trick. A woman wants to feel you are present with her during an intimate session. Clear any doubts and arouse her by breathing softly into her ears.

Back

The back of a woman is generally less sensitive to touch, but don't ignore it. You just need to deepen your touch on this area. The sacral curve, just above a woman's buttocks, is more sensitive than other parts of the back. Take time to massage, touch, kiss and rub this region for intense relaxation and stimulation. Lower back touching also helps to ease your way into other more sensitive areas such as the groin and buttocks.

Buttocks

Some women might not be comfortable to show their buttocks. Communicate to determine her comfort level. If she is open to it, buttocks touching can help her reach another level of sexual excitement. As partners, you must have a mutual understanding of how this area is handled.

Breasts

Men love breasts. However, this area must be touched sparingly. Yes, you heard me correctly. Most men spend too much time on the breasts and they forget to touch other areas. True breasts are a very sensitive part of a woman and that when touched correctly, can relax and arouse her. But don't fixate on them. Explore other areas of her body too. More than on her breasts, place a hand in the middle of her chest and hold it, making her feel like you're there with her. That you are not in a hurry and that you are walking together towards the same place.

Hair

Touching and playing with your partner's hair is intimate and exciting. It can also be incredibly soothing. Begin with a few kisses, and then gently touch her beautiful locks. Lift her hair just enough to reveal her neck and plant kisses on her neck all the way up to her hairline. You can also gentle rub her head or simply place your lips against it. Your breath warmly penetrating her hair onto her head is relaxing, intimate, and arousing.

Face

To successfully relax your partner as well as to maximize foreplay with her, you cannot forget the face. Start with your fingers, gently touching her from her lips, to her ears, nose, eyes, cheeks, and chin. Then use your tongue or lips along the same path. Do this with great care. Attend to the face carefully for safety, optimal relaxation, and ultimate stimulation.

Limbs

Do not forget a woman's hands, arms, wrists, feet, and legs. Touch them. Kiss them. Lick them. Rub them. Moving out to the tips of her body connects you to every inch of her, reducing stress, increasing relaxation and strengthening your bond as a couple.

The gist of it is: Understand your partner; know her body like your own; learn what she wants and how she wants it. Sex should be mutual: mutually relaxing and mutually rewarding. Communicate with your partner to understand all the whats, wheres and hows of relaxing her and turning her on. By so doing, sex will not be such hard work, but rather full of excitement and satisfaction.

A More Intimate Touch

To explore your partner's body and uncover what she loves, your fingers and hands play a vital role. We will explore some ways to use your hands (and of course communication) during foreplay and sex.

Hygiene is very important. Always make sure your hands are clean before touching a woman's sensitive areas. In order to create optimal sexual excitement in your partner, you must know where to touch or stimulate first. While some women prefer to be stimulated on the clitoris first, others prefer being touched on the vulva. Either way, it is advised that you make use of a lubricant to keep the woman wet all throughout the session. Pay attention to your partner's movement. She will often guide you by moving in the direction she wants to be touched.

It is not difficult to discover how your partner loves to be touched in respect to motion, the intensity of pressure, or speed. Below are three recommendations for intimate touching.

1. Begin by placing your palm on the area where her pubic hair begins and exert pressure. Rest your hands, which you have lubricated, on her labia with your finger facing her anus.

2. Try touching her outer and inner lips with your thumb and forefinger. This should be done gently. Continue exerting pressure with your palm on her pubic hair area while carefully moving your fingers in circles. Be careful not to move randomly over her skin. Start with slow movements then gradually increase your pace.

3. Continue with this motion until you have moved your

fingers for at least eight rounds. After this, you can move your fingers to her vagina and give her gentle taps, at least eight times.

4. Repeat the whole process from the top for as long as you and your partner desire.

5. Then, stop, and leave your hand on his intimate area and breathe together.

6. Pay attention to the heat emitted from the area in question and the possible micromovements that may occur.

7. Thinning your sensitivity, you may come to notice by placing your index finger at the entrance of the vulva, which will be the one through the internal spasms that will suck your finger into it.

Chapter 6:

The Point of No Return

These words describe the stage you get to when you can no longer keep yourself from ejaculating from the passionate and irrepressible session of sexual arousal.

To help you go longer without climaxing, you will have to learn to slow down when you feel yourself build up to that point. Take a deep breath, to ensure you dissipate that built up energy as much as you can to prolong your experience.

What does the point of no return feel like? Here are a few things that are happening when you near that point.

- Passion is becoming the master of your will and an attempt to subdue your feelings becomes more difficult.

- Then your command over your sexual performance and your body begins to decrease.

- You are becoming subordinate to self-indulgence and sensations.

- Here you are feeling hyper-stimulated, as indicated by your rapid, shallow breathing and frantic motions. Less morally inclined people may display profanity, become quite rude or offensive, and unfortunately could also become physically abusive with their partner.

- The male organ heats up.

- There comes a feeling of bliss and an unmistakable inability to think straight. This feeling has been likened by many men to being under the influence of alcohol.

- A thrill runs down your spine settling in your genital area.

- Your profound thrusts illustrate your raised need for speed and eagerness for passionate expression. Your command over your body is greatly reduced.

- You can't miss the exciting tremors beginning to manifest at this point, and when they come, you can be sure that your climax is just around the corner.

- Alas, you have just had an orgasm.

All of the above can happen as a low build up or quickly, giving you no time to react appropriately. Either way, you can always see and feel it coming if you are attentive enough.

By paying close attention to your body and these signals we can avoid the point of no return and rapid ejaculation.

What to Do When You Realize the Point of No Return is Close?

1. Pause. Take a couple of minutes during which you loosen up and let all the pent-up energy dissipate through the rest of your body.

2. If after the pause you still don't feel less tense and still feel ready to spill, then you should withdraw and then perform this easy trick to help you dissipate the energy:

   — Contract and relax the sphincters of your anus.

   — Do the same for the pelvic floor.

3. Loosen up and let your whole pelvis relax and feel the pent-up energy reverse back up your spine and dissipate through your body. Before you know it, you are back in command of your body and it's safe to proceed.

If you are worried about how your partner will feel during these techniques, then you can do it covertly.

I know that at the beginning it may seem strange to you to carry out these preventive techniques, especially if you do it in front of your partner. But I assure you that when she understands that the focus you're doing this for and being able to give both of you more pleasure, these techniques will become an integral part of your new couple games.

These easy techniques don't have to be done on "special occasions." In fact, it is advisable to incorporate them into your usual routine for managing PE.

You can try them anywhere: on the bus, in a meeting, while

driving, walking—*anywhere.* In addition to improving your sexual control these exercises can also have positive effects on your frame of mind and overall morale.

If you are a man who recently became sexually active or are someone who gets aroused very easily, then it is advisable that you go on much longer pauses. You might even consider including using a cold shower to cool off your penis. Do not use this cooling method for more than five minutes.

Having a very understanding and patient partner will come in handy at this stage of your journey as you learn to take control over your sexual performance and health. Without communication and a compassionate partner, this stage of your life might prove difficult and frustrating. But you can do it! I know you can do it because you are now aware of all the signals of the point of no return and the simple tricks and techniques that will help you to avoid a premature orgasm. You can be confident that you are gradually becoming a master of your sexual energy.

Chapter 7:

The PC Muscle

One of the muscles that make up the human pelvic floor is the pubococcygeus muscle (PC). It spreads from the tailbone (coccyx) to the pubic bone. The PC muscle holds the genitals on the inside.

The muscle is responsible for bowel control, urine continence, and urine release. It is also what makes an erect penis bob up and down on its own. One of its most essential functions, with respect to this topic, is its role in orgasms and ejaculation. Even for women, the OC muscle intensifies sensation, climaxes, and excitation during sex.

You can easily assess your PC muscle control during urination. Even though you can't necessarily feel it with your hands, you can feel it while urinating. Try halting your urination midstream or squeeze those final drops out. The muscle responsible for these that you're feeling work is the PC muscle.

You can test out the development of your PC muscle by contracting the muscles at the base of your erect organ to make it bob up and down. Your muscle is developed if you can keep your muscle contracted for at least 20 seconds and for 25 times in a row.

Knowing that the PC muscle is responsible for ejaculation and understanding the workings of the PC muscle may just be your saving grace. Do not underestimate the significance of the PC muscle. Find your PC muscle, feel its movement, observe your control, and then try to be more in control of it to improve how long you can spend in bed.

Failure to understand your PC muscle will keep you from

developing its strength. A limp PC muscle can cause:

- The inability to assess how aroused you are during intercourse and thereby leaving you unprepared and more likely to experience premature ejaculation

- Powerless ejaculations without force and good texture

- A frustrating time just trying to stay 'hard'

- The need to have a long recovery time after climaxing, lengthening the time before the next intercourse

Exercising the PC Muscle

The strength of your PC muscles is crucial in having or not having a great sex life. Many men under this tutelage have increased their sexual experience by practicing the exercises below for only 10 minutes over the span of a week.

The majority of the techniques can be done anywhere and anytime without anyone being the wiser. You don't have to take off your clothes or expose your genitals. All you need is a little concentration.

It is essential that you do these exercises in your own time and at your own speed. Don't rush the process or stress yourself. Just follow the instructions and you will feel and see the positive changes.

Kegel Exercises for Men

Just like women, men can do Kegel exercises too. The exercises reinforce the sturdiness of the muscles making up the pelvic floor.

Exercising the pelvic floor routinely is known to help both PE and erectile dysfunction. You can combine medications with your Kegel exercises for your treatment of PE. Like all exercise, don't expect to see the results of Kegels instantaneously. Dedication and commitment will produce good results in time.

Locate your pelvic floor muscles

Before you can exercise your pelvic muscles, you first have to find them. Loosen up any tension in your thigh muscles, abdomen, and butt.

Contract the muscles around your anus like you would do when you are trying hard not to fart, after which you can relax them. Do this alternatively till you are certain that you have targeted the accurate muscles. Be sure that while you tense your anal muscles, you don't contract your butt or the abdominal muscles.

There is also a trick to help you locate your penile glans (to target the urethra). Contract like you would when trying to stop urine in mid-stream. If you get it right, then you will see and feel your penis withdraw a little into your pelvis. Next time you go to the bathroom to urinate, try out the movement, and note the muscles affected to ensure you are on the right track.

Exercise the muscles of your pelvic floor

Having learned how to find the muscles making up the pelvic floor, you can move on to your Kegel exercises. You can alternate between fast Kegel exercises and slow Kegel exercises. In all these exercises the most important thing will be the degree of cohesion between muscle movement and breathing. Once you have learned to manage and control the ejaculatory moment, it is only through your breath that you will be able to learn how to manipulate and use the energy not dissipated when you do not come. You will experience what is called internal ejaculation.

Slow Kegels

- Squeeze the muscles that make up the pelvic floor for

five seconds, let go for another five seconds. Don't forget to breathe!

- Do the contraction and relaxation technique again, being very deliberate and slow. You can work towards repeating this 10 times.

- If you ever feel discomfort while doing these contractions, stop and rest.

- The more you work at it, the more you should aim for. Try a longer hold beyond five seconds. Don't forget to hold your contractions and relaxations for the same amount of time.

Fast Kegels

- Follow the same Kegel techniques as you do in slow Kegels: You are doing the same thing (squeeze, hold, let go) with some time adjustments.

- In fast Kegels, you reduce the length of time of the contractions and rest periods. Hold for about one second, let go, and then go again almost immediately.

- Alternate between fast and slow Kegels after a set of 10 reps each.

- As time goes on, raise the number of reps from 10 to 15 to 20 and so on.

Maximum Kegel

- Sit on the edge of a chair, avoiding sofas and armchairs that are too soft.

- Position yourself with your legs slightly apart and place your hands on your knees to ensure more stability in your position.

- Bring your thumbs inside your hand.

- Tighten the muscles that make up the pelvic floor, trying to include the muscles that surround the anal area as well. (In this exercise we look for the longest contraction we can maintain).

- Make a slow and deep inhalation as soon as the contraction starts.

- Keep your breathing and contraction as much as possible.

- Exhale and relax the stressed muscles, very slowly.

- Start with 3 sets of ten repetitions.

Timed stimulation

In this exercise you will need a stopwatch or a simple clock to mark the seconds.

- Sit on the edge of a chair, avoiding sofas and armchairs that are too soft.

- Position yourself with your legs slightly apart and place your hands on your knees to ensure more stability in your position.

- Bring your thumbs inside your hand.

- Tighten the muscles that make up the pelvic floor and release the contraction.
- This time the exercise should be done at maximum speed. That is, short and quick contractions.

- The exercise consists of performing the maximum amount of repetitions that your body allows you, in a period of time of one minute. Try to count your contractions.

- Do the exercise at least 3 times.

Do not give too much importance to breathing in this exercise. If you are just starting out, it will be impossible to administer the logistics of these three motor functions (contraction, breathing, counting).

- As the days go by, check the results.

A constant and routine execution of these exercises will lead you in a short time to duplicate the results of the first days. Have confidence.
On average, the results for neophytes of this in this world range from 35 to 55 contractions per minute. Don't worry about whatever your initial number of contractions is, just try to exceed your limit with your training.

How often should you practice Kegel exercises?

The simple answer is: as often as possible. Kegel exercises are recommended three to five times daily, but if you can do more, do it! Time shouldn't be a constraint, as five sets of 10 fast Kegel reps will take you under a minute. The most time you should be spending, however, is 10 minutes a day. Set a starting goal for yourself of at least three sets of both fast and slow Kegels every day.

However committed you might be, it's always easy to forget. Try to fix your Kegel time in easy-to-remember periods throughout the day. Here are some suggestions as to when to exercise:

- One of the first things you do in the morning, just after waking up

- After going to the bathroom

- While driving to work

- Before, during, or after your lunch break

- One of the last things you do just before you go to sleep

Whatever time you choose, make it regular. Once you have incorporated Kegels into your daily routine, you can try it during intercourse.

Chapter 8:

Breathing

You will notice if you are attentive enough during sex that your breathing is usually all over the place, rapid and shallow at some stage and slow and deep at another stage. Sometimes, you may even find your nose inadequate in your breathing process and you find that soon to your horror that your mouth is hanging open.

Awareness is essential in the fight against PE. So be aware of everything, including your breathing, during every stage of intercourse. This way, you can retrace your steps and pinpoint the root of an issue.

Breathing affects the heart rate, and subsequently, your excitement. You can see this in the stage of arousal when men start breathing fast and shallow with the consequence of hyperstimulation.

Be deliberate about breathing slowly and deeply after every three to four seconds. It may prove uneasy at first, but keep at it. Whether you breathe through your mouth or nose, keep it slow and deep. Try to keep the same intervals of three to four seconds throughout.

Practice is the key to this. With enough practice and attention maintaining in your controlled breaths, over time, will become natural, and you'll be a master of your breathing. The relationship between breathing, excitation and climax is strong. If you can command your breathing, then you can command your libido and your climax moment.

Being aware of your breathing enough to know when to slow it down, increase it or just breathe normally can help you last longer in bed. If you are aware and can effectively make the changes in your breathing for you to perform better and longer. Here are a few specific breathing exercises to get you on your way.

Breathing Exercise 1

Don't underestimate the strong adverse effects of anxiety. No matter how accurately you follow the steps, how well you have mastered your breathing, or how often you practice your Kegel exercises, if you are anxious during intercourse, everything you have worked for will crumble before your eyes as you ejaculate prematurely yet again!

Take deep breaths. As you take deep breaths, feel your diaphragm expand as your ribs descend. Breathing through your upper chest will only cause limitations in breathing so while taking that deep breath, ensure you can feel the descent of your diaphragm. This will help you relax, and abate anxiety making you last longer and perform better.

Studies have shown that these breathing techniques promote vitality and stamina during intercourse. Making it a habit to breathe deeply and from your diaphragm will help you learn to regulate your orgasms as opposed to breathing from the chest, which only expends energy and makes you anxious.

Breathe in slowly and steadily via the nose and breathe out through the mouth. Shut your eyes while taking in air through the nose. With every breath you take, focus on your breathing. Don't get too fixated on the pleasure you are getting from the intercourse and forget your breathing.

After inhaling and holding for about five seconds, exhale very slowly. Do it, again and again, every 15 to 40 seconds. The exact number of seconds in between is determined by how grim your case of premature ejaculation is.

This exercise is not just simple, but it is also very productive. With this exercise, you can be tranquil and collected while still feeling pleasure from the sexual experience.

Breathing Exercise 2

This exercise is as simple to carry out and as effective as the first exercise in prolonging your sexual experience. It can be practiced while masturbating but is most recommended while having intercourse with your partner. It's done by withdrawing your penis while inhaling and thrusting it while exhaling. While practicing this technique, you still need to simultaneously focus on your deep and slow breathing. You can try this technique every four to eight penetrations.

You can train your body and your mind to learn sweet restraint by penetrating with deliberate thrusts and breathing. This coupling is essential to your sexual performance and comes in handy for much of what you've learned and will learn in this book.

Chapter 9:

The Squeeze Technique

In this technique, the phallus is squeezed using the thumb and index finger just before the man's orgasm. This action somewhat decreases the intensity of his erection and consequently prolongs his stamina.

There have been several claims that this technique has worked for men with PE in incredible ways. I admit, however, that the technique requires lots of practice in order to master it. You need to think about the perfect squeeze spot, ideal pressure with which to squeeze, and most importantly: the timing. Several men involve their women by letting them do the squeezing. Research and studies have shown that there is an incredible effect the technique has on men with PE but after proper search on literature review was conducted, it was found out that the studies and research carried out have not been done formally.

This technique comes in two parts. Mastering the first part of the technique is most important.

How to Perform the Squeeze Techniques

Part 1: Mastering the squeeze technique

1. You need to get fully erect. You can involve your partner in this.

2. After obtaining a full erection, place a thumb (yours or your partner's) on the frenulum, which is a strip of skin just between the head and the prepuce of the penis.

3. Now, place your index and middle digits on the dorsal part of the penis just opposite the thumb's position.

4. Check to make sure that the index and middle digits are near one another but on either side of the coronal ridge (the little ridge just by the tip, a few centimeters away from the very top).

5. Lastly, you can squeeze all placed fingers on the penis together for about four seconds and squeeze firmly. Your partner may not know how hard to squeeze so you might have to help her by squeezing with her till she gets the hang of it.

6. Pause for at most 30 seconds before letting go of the penis. It is normal to not be as erect after the squeezing.

7. After being stimulated to a state of full erection again, repeat the process about four more times.

8. Then proceed with the intercourse and try to maintain your control over ejaculation.

Part 2: Ejaculatory control using the squeeze technique

1. Stimulate yourself until you are near a climax.

2. Practice the squeeze technique.

3. Don't forget to time the squeezing carefully. If you feel like you are fast approaching orgasm too soon after you start again, then you most probably missed the timing and squeezed a bit too late. It might take several sessions to get it right, but you will.

4. Repeat about four more times, but don't let the whole process take away from the pleasure of copulating with your partner or the anticipated mind-blowing orgasm.

5. You can progress on to practicing the same technique using oral sex.

6. Now practice time is over. It's time for the real deal: vaginal sex.

7. During intercourse, use the technique at least a couple times before the actual penetration, perhaps while engaging in foreplay.

Chapter 10:

Meditation for Premature Ejaculation

Meditation is a powerful tool in analyzing your thoughts, emotions, and affections. It enables you to "step out of yourself" as though in the third person.

The practice of meditation enhances one's ability to gain control over their mind and maintain stable mental awareness. Consistent practice will enable you to get acquainted with your thoughts. It will also give you the capacity to take charge of your physical feelings.

The practice of meditation helps individuals suffering from premature ejaculation gain control over it. When you practice the art of meditation in the right way, it will help you gain mental control over your sexual arousal and put you in full control of ejaculation.

You are most likely to lose control over what is going on in your mind if your mind is always "on the move." This can cause the rapid snowball of worries and anxieties.

To allow your mind to function well, there is a great need for you to consciously and intentionally stop the thoughts going on inside of it, regard this as a process of mental housekeeping.

Allow the spinning thoughts in your mind to reduce their pace. Eventually, they will automatically come to a halt. This will put you at the center of control while you still have a grip on your consciousness.

It is imperative to examine every thought and never let your emotions get out of control. This will transform everything about you, including your life in the bedroom.

Keeping your mind calm and away from any form of arousing factors, such as porn, will enable you to masturbate as long as you want and as hard as you want without ejaculating. Meditation helps you to put your mind in this calm almost blank state while masturbating.

Meditation during your passionate throes of lovemaking is a lot more difficult than when it is just between you and your own hands.

Nevertheless, if you can successfully equip your mind with the skill of meditation during the process of masturbating, it will be much easier for you to effectively use the skill during sexual intercourse.

Below are some of the many Yoga techniques that will allow you to revitalize your body, become aware of it and reinvigorate your sexual energy. In each of the following techniques, the fundamental part will always be breathing. Breathing represents the bridge that connects you with your Higher Self, with your deepest consciousness.
If there are any doubts regarding the description of the positions to be performed, I invite you to look on youtube how to perform them. The information material available online is endless to say the least, and the funniest thing is that it's free. Take advantage!

Sarvanga Asana

This asana aids in revitalizing the whole body system. It facilitates the smooth running of the thyroid gland, which serves as a catalyst in enabling the work of bodily functions (The Health Site, 2015). After doing this asana, I realised that it increased my metabolism, making me energetic and vitalized throughout the day. It helps in giving more strength and agility to the adrenal glands, enhancing the testes, and ultimately increasing the potency of the semen and sperm (Jain, 2017).

Procedures to carry out this pose

- Spread a yoga mat on the floor and lie flat with your legs shooting outwards.

- Raise your legs up. You can raise them by folding your legs at the knees or by slowly lifting them straight.

- Put your palms around your and hips to support your position.

- Lift your buttocks and back off the mat with your toes pointing upwards with your elbows firmly held on your back and pressed to the floor. By this time, the weight of your body should be on your shoulders.

- Lock your chin into your chest and breathe slowly. Stay in this position for as long as you can, when tired, slowly return to lying position.

Under no circumstances should you embark on this exercise if you suffer from neck pain or spinal injuries.

If you are a patient of high blood pressure, make sure you are under supervision while doing this. In any case, it is always best to ask a doctor about your physical capabilities and restrictions before practicing.

Uttanapadasana

This exercise is solely aimed at strengthening the intestines. According to Ayurvedic principles, the intestine is an important organ for maintaining a healthy body.

It wasn't as easy doing this pose. You might have to do this under the supervision of a trained expert, especially if you suffer from knee or back pain.

This asana has diverse benefits. It helps to defeat constipation, increases one's metabolism, and fights digestion problems. It is also believed that it can help a man defeat premature ejaculation (The Health Site, 2015; Jain, 2017).

Procedures to carry out this pose

- Lie flat on a yoga mat with your facing the ceiling.

- Position your heels together and place your hands by your side.

- Lift your head and legs off the ground to a 30-degree position. Remain there for a couple of seconds, and then slowly return to lying position.

- Take a deep breath then raise your legs again, this time to a 60-degree position.

- Hold for a few seconds then release. If you discover that lifting both legs up at the same time is too difficult, start with one at a time until you are stronger and more flexible.

Kandharasana

This asana facilitates the sexual desire of both men and women. It also strengthens the abilities of the male's sperm, which helps to reduce infertility (The Health Site, 2015; Jain, 2017). When I tried this pose I observed that it improved my rate of breathing.

Procedures to carry out this pose

- Lie flat on a yoga mat; bend your knees until your ankles are touching your butt. Make sure that your legs are separated.

- Hold your ankles while still lying down.

- Breathe in and hold your breath in that position.

- Slowly raise your buttocks in the air and press your chest towards the ceiling. Your back must be curved and off the floor. Remain in this position for as long as you can.

- Breathe out and lie back down to return to your normal position.

Make sure are supervised by a trained expert if you suffer from lower back pain, a spinal disorder or high blood pressure.

Paschimot Asana

This is arguably one of the best asanas to defeat premature ejaculation. It makes the semen more potent, which helps in resolving infertility. It also helps boost the metabolism (Jain, 2017). I have recommended this to a few friends, and it not only helped them last in bed, it also improved their digestive issues.

Procedures to carry out this pose

- Sit on a yoga mat with your legs stretched out on the floor.

- Breathe out and slowly bend pressing your head towards your knees.

- Hold your toes with your index fingers and thumbs.

- Be careful to not let your elbows touch the ground. While holding your breath, remain in this position for a few seconds.

- When you start to feel uncomfortable, breath in as you return to the sitting position.

This exercise is not suitable for individuals that have any form of back or spinal pain. Also, do not be too hard on yourself. My friends were not able to get their forehead to touch their knees in the first attempt. However, consistent practice helped their flexibility and enabled them to eventually do the pose correctly.

Goumukhasana

This is a pose that comes with a wide range of benefits. It is known to treat hernias and hydrolysis disorder, a condition where fluid builds up in the testes region. It also helps to prevent premature ejaculation and revitalize the liver, kidney, and respiratory system (Dhikav, Karmarkar, Gupta & Anand, 2007; Jain, 2017).

Procedures to carry out this pose

- You can do this asana while in a kneeling position on your yoga mat putting the upper part of the body in a vertical position while balancing your weight on your knees. Those with a knee injury or arthritis can take a seat in padmasana pose to be able to do this. Ensure your toes are reaching for the ground

- Form a curve by warping your right hand and positioning it at your back. Ensure the edges of your fingers are leaning upwards near the spinal column.

- Place your left hand over your head warping, carefully passing to the backside of your collar region and interlock with your right hand. Hold for a few seconds, then try inhaling and exhaling through the pose.

- Sit down and return your hands to their normal positions.

You must remember that at first you may not have the ability to stretch your hands completely together. I also found this difficult in my first attempt, but not to worry. It will get better with constant practice and you will soon be as flexible as a newborn baby.

Bhujangasana

This asana can help premature ejaculation and improve longevity in bed. It can also be used as a remedy for a sore back and neck pain (Dhikav, Karmarkar, Gupta & Anand, 2007; Jain, 2017).

Procedures to carry out this pose

- Lie down horizontally on your belly; both your head and your feet should be touching the floor.

- Position both your hands on the floor next to your shoulders with your elbows pointing out.

- Breathe out and raise the upper part of your body gradually starting from the head, then moving on to lifting the chest, back, and pelvis.

- Afterwards, relax your body, still lying on your belly; however, ensure both hands are still together with no space between the elbows. Then balance on both hands evenly with your belly still touching the floor's surface.

- Clear your mind while inhaling and exhaling.

- Finish the pose by exhaling and return to your initial position of lying flat on the floor. You can come to a sitting position by using your palms for balance.

This is my favorite pose when I'm feeling depressed and it also helped me with PE. If you have a wrist injury or a sore back, please do not do this pose.

Dhanur Asana

This asana serves as a remedy to premature ejaculation, helps to cure stomach disorders and can also be used to increase orgasms (Dhikav, Karmarkar, Gupta & Anand, 2007).

Procedures to carry out this pose

- Lie flat on the floor or yoga mat on your belly, slightly spread your feet apart from the hips and place your hands beside your body.

- Bend your knees and carefully grasp your ankles with both hands.

- While breathing in, raise the upper part of your body from the floor surface and gently push the lower part of your body upwards and backwards.

- Keep your breathing normal and your position steady with positive energy radiating from the face (a smile).

- Maintain your position for as long as you can whilst watching your breathing. Stretch at a moderate level that your body can handle. You don't want to overstretch your muscles on the first go.

- To finish the pose, carefully place your lower and upper body back on the floor, and remove your hands from your ankles.

People suffering from a hernia, cervical pain, back pain, abnormal blood pressure, headache, and pregnant women or those recovering from abdominal surgery should refrain from doing this pose.

Brahmachary Asana

This asana is perfect for people with premature ejaculation and a low libido. It helps to increase libido and sexual prowess and improve the functioning of the testes and digestive system (Dhikav, Karmarkar, Gupta & Anand, 2007; Jain, 2017).

Procedures to carry out this pose

- Sit on your knees. Spreading your feet away from each other with your knees together.

- Gently lower your upper body backward in the gap between your knee and feet.

- Put your palms on your knees, towards the floor and keep track of your breathing.

- Close your eyes to help you stay focused on the pose for a few minutes.

- Finish the pose by raising your upper body from the gap and closing your knees.

This pose has a lot to do with the knees. I have tried it a few times and can feel that you should not participate in this pose if you suffer from a knee injury.

Garud Asana

This asana suppresses the negative effects of reproductive diseases while also benefiting the urinary tract, testes, and prostate gland. It also serves as a remedy to premature ejaculation (Dhikav, Karmarkar, Gupta & Anand, 2007; Jain, 2017).

Procedures to carry out this pose

- Position yourself by standing on your yoga mat, shifting your body weight to your right leg.

- Bend your right leg, slightly raise and place your left leg around your right leg. This should leave your left foot touching your right heel.

- Lift your hands up to your face level, fingers pointing up and elbows bent.

- Next, place your right elbow in the fold of your left elbow. Wrap your hands so they are interlocking. Your palms should be together.

- Maintain the position for a few seconds and then return to Tadasana to finish the pose.

In the beginning, you might not be able to maintain your pose for a prolonged period but don't worry. This asana requires constant practice and focus.

Anulom Vilom Pranayama

Anulom Vilom Pranayama is a breathing technique that is used for curing coughs, colds, respiratory allergies, sinusitis, and rhinitis (inflammation of the nasal cavity). It can also be used to increase sexual prowess and longevity in bed (Mamidi & Gupta, 2013).

Procedures to carry out this pose

- Sit on a mat with your knees completely folded into a padmasana pose. Bend your legs as much as you can if you find it difficult to fold them completely.

- Place one hand forwards ensuring your palm is facing upwards.

- Fold the index finger of the free hand, and place the thumb of the same free hand on one nostril.

- Extend the ring finger to be sure it can reach the second nostril. To avoid weakening your elbow, leave it low and loose on your side.

- Deeply breathe through one nostril keeping the second nostril closed every time you breathe in through it. Invert the process, closing the first nostril and breathing in through the second. This completes one cycle.

- Repeat this cycle, starting with three minutes and gradually increasing it to around 15 to 20 minutes.

- While breathing in, it is not recommended to slouch. Also ensure your breaths are deep, and through your lungs, so that your stomach isn't filled with air.

Keep in mind when practicing these poses that Yoga is all about posture and patience. It is not an exercise that you can rush through. When I tried this pose I noticed I needed to work on my strength and balance. Take time to learn the postures correctly and focus less on duration if needed. In Yoga always stay calm, breathe normally and align your body with your mind.

Chapter 11:

Loving Yourself

To Love Another, You Must First Love Yourself

A healthy relationship is one where both parties are comfortable and happy with one another. But first, each partner must be happy with his or herself before love can grow and overflow to others.

Most individuals are too scared to accept their flaws so we end up falling in love for all the wrong reasons. For example, some get into a relationship simply to counter loneliness, to ease pain, or to seek comfort. However, true happiness comes from working on yourself to become the person you wish to be.

Change, they say, is the only constant thing in life and self-growth can encourage such changes. Self-growth promotes self-awareness, and realistic and healthy aspirations.

No one has gained complete mastery of this instantly. We only learn to cope with our problems by pressing forward, no matter what comes our way, don't allow your past to affect your future and how you view yourself.

Your happiness is in your hands and it's up to you to make sure you're happy. Worry less about your life's problems and learn how to make yourself smile.

My advice on this is:

Stop criticizing yourself all the time

"Don't worry if others don't like you. Worry if you don't appreciate yourself."

Confucius.

No one is perfect, we are here to learn and evolve. Instead of pointing your finger at every mistake you make, try to hold out your arm and move on. To make a mistake is human, with every mistake, learn to improve next time. These words may seem obvious to you, but that's all there is to know.
And remember that your intent is to build a solid foundation within you, not to demolish it.

Stop comparing yourself to others

"When you're happy to just be yourself and don't compare and don't compete, everyone will respect you."

Lao Tzu

You are unique! No one can ever be like you, and you can never be someone else.   Observing others will take

energy away from you and your goals, distracting you from the only person with whom it makes sense to compete: yourself.
The more you focus on discovering yourself, the more you will feel like knowing what others are doing. Don't waste precious time!

Don't identify yourself by the context in which you live

"To have that sense of one's own intrinsic value that constitutes self-respect is to have potentially everything."

Joan Didion

Society continuously places us in categories, for which most of the time with the passing of time we begin to identify ourselves. I'm sorry, but I'm not here! If it were the way society wants it, this example should be certain, right? That is, I do a prestigious job, so I am a prestigious person. As well as (on the contrary): I do a small job, I am a small person. Well, I hope you've all understood what I mean. You're a lot more than you do. You've spent your whole life hearing yourself say where you should look. First you had to look to the right, then to the left, forward or backward. Has anyone ever taught you to look inside yourself? That's where your best part resides.

Learn to say NO

When you say "yes" to someone, make sure you don't say "no" to yourself.

(Anonymous)

In other words, learn to say NO without falling into the temptation to please others at all costs. The message that you are more or less consciously communicating by always agreeing to everything and everyone is something like, "I'm not worth enough, and I need your approval to finally feel considered and loved. You have to honor your authenticity and this sometimes also means taking responsibility for disagreement with someone. Remember that saying NO doesn't mean you want to argue at all. Maybe it's because of your NO that you'll find out how to do something better!

I know that for most men, saying therapist would be a bit like blaspheming! Rest assured. Let me explain. Let me give you an example. You have a problem with your car, maybe it's a flat tire. What do you do? Do you go to a mechanic to repair it or do you keep going around the city as if nothing had happened... at the cost of causing further damage to the car? This is one of the problems of us men. We don't feel like men if we ask for help! Peace to their souls. I asked for help when I needed it, and now, this allowed me to help myself first and other people in turn. We are here in this life, not to demonstrate but to learn. Do this, don't go to a Therapist, consult a Sex-coach, maybe calling it that way will make you feel less uncomfortable!

Most often, we focus only on getting what we want now and less about the future. We must learn to enjoy the present and live in it rather than seeing it as a way of escaping loneliness or filling a void.

Filling the void only brings temporary relief, but satisfying our emotional needs can do much more. Unfortunately, it also requires more effort.

Therefore, you need to create your own happiness and learn to manage your personal issues. In addition, create opportunities and a lifestyle that gives you control over your happiness. Focus on changes that drive you and make you feel blessed. At times, you might find yourself in a situation in which you may need to change significantly and it's likely time to let go of some behaviors.

Usually, we attempt to fix the scars of others by subscribing to the idea that love heals all pain. But you need to recover from your own wounds before attempting to fix those of the other person.

True, there is no perfect relationship; however, there is a thin line between settling for less because it makes you feel happy now and denying the reality of your potential. Don't live with regrets; rather, focus on the lessons you learned from the past.

Dig Deep

Did you know that you attract what you are? You meet someone new and immediately you feel so drawn to that person because both of you just seem to understand each other and the chemistry can't be explained. Can you ever ignore such instant, magnetic connections? Like you, I find these feelings difficult to ignore.

Simply put, if you're amazing, you'll attract amazing people. And if you're a crappy individual, you'll attract a person like that. If you focus on working on your problems not only will you attract a better person, you will also improve yourself in the meantime. Plus, few things bring as much joy and satisfaction as looking in the rearview mirror of your life to see how far you've come.

When seeking a relationship, go for one in which both partners have independently discovered themselves rather than trying to discover yourself through the other person. You need to dig deep within to discover yourself and your self-worth. Staying single and happy is way better than being stuck in an unhappy relationship.

Being in a relationship should not reflect some sort of dependency on the other person. Rather, it should be a demonstration of the strength of togetherness. Be extremely cautious while trying to decide the person you will give your heart to. Your happiness should be a matter of choice, not chance. Since happiness is an independent state of mind, only you hold the keys to your happiness, so be aware of whom you allow access into your life.

Loving Yourself Can Enhance Your Sex Life

A man's mood can affect his eating habits and his sex life. Everything is directly linked to self-esteem and body image. If you hate yourself, you will likely experience eating problems, challenges in the bedroom, or both. Extraordinary is how love for oneself and food are bound. One influences the other and vice versa. Do you want a change in your life? Start with food. Love your body, give yourself the pleasure of preparing succulent healthy dishes. If your belly, stomach is happy, so will your head, your mind. I don't say it, the doctors say it. Then, add some physical activity during the week, and that's where you'll want to write a book about how your life has changed! Coming back to us, a man with little self-esteem will prefer to undress in the dark because he feels he is not attractive enough, he won't be able to last long enough, or he might ejaculate too soon. Such a man will not fully enjoy sex and may feel he does not deserve to be loved. That's why I push you to get involved, to push yourself beyond what you thought were your limits. Society is very good at giving you a label, putting you in a category and leaving you there your whole life. Don't let them if you don't like it. If you feel uncomfortable, where you are right now, you break the chains that immobilize you, and you take charge of your life. Study, inform and keep your body trained. "Mens sana in corpore sano", make your body your Temple.

Is Poor Self-Image Affecting Your Sex Life?

A man with poor self-esteem will prefer to undress in the dark because he feels he's not big enough, he won't be able to hold on long enough, or might ejaculate too soon. Such a man will not enjoy sex fully and might feel he doesn't deserve to be loved.

Building Self-Love

If you feel your self-perception is negatively impacting your ability to fully enjoy sex, maybe it's time for some self-love. You need to review the reasons why you feel that way and try to find ways to break that wall in your mind. With the help of a skilled therapist, this process can become much easier.

I know that for most men, saying therapist would be a bit like blaspheming! Rest assured. Let me explain. Let me give you an example. You have a problem with your car, maybe it's a flat tire. What do you do? Do you go to a mechanic to repair it or do you keep going around the city as if nothing had happened... at the cost of causing further damage to the car?

This is one of the problems of us men. We don't feel like men if we ask for help! Peace to their souls. I asked for help when I needed it, and now, this allowed me to help myself first and other people in turn. We are here in this life, not to demonstrate but to learn. Do this, don't go to a Therapist, consult a Sex-coach, maybe calling it that way will make you feel less uncomfortable!

Becoming Connected With Your Body

In order to experience pleasurable sex, your body, heart, and genitals need to be in tune with each other. However, obsessive feelings could bring about a disconnection and all the pleasure will be lost. To enjoy sex, you need to shut your mind from all distractions, and focus all of your attention on yourself and the person in the bedroom. Let go of all the distracting thoughts in your mind and take a dive into the space in your heart. Ask yourself: What do I feel? What shapes and colors do I see? What does my heart want? Master this self-talk and you can use it anytime.

Though the path to self-acceptance is usually a long one, taking this a bold step is worth the effort. It can help you overcome self-hatred and improve your sex life in more ways than you can imagine.

Chapter 12:

Consider a Prescription

There are certain drugs that can help PE. One of them is antidepressants. Antidepressants that target PE are the selective serotonin reuptake inhibitors (SSRIs). The whole mechanism of ejaculation is regulated by two chemical messengers or 'neurotransmitters', dopamine, and serotonin.

While dopamine reduces the threshold for ejaculation thereby initiating ejaculation, serotonin prolongs the experience and holds back a climax by increasing the threshold for ejaculation (Waldinger *et al.*, 2005). Hence these SSRIs help to regulate the levels of neurotransmitters. Men with PE are known to have a reduced amount of serotonin in their blood.

Basically, SSRIs help to elongate the time you have sex before climaxing by raising your serotonin levels, thereby raising your ejaculation threshold and Intravaginal Ejaculatory Latency Time (IELT). I suggest not getting your hopes too high because it may not work in such a spectacular and simple way for everyone. But if you have severe PE, then it might be worth a try.

Think of the drugs not as a remedy but rather as an integral part of your scheme to get rid of PE. It's best to follow this line of thought because drugs in themselves will not procure a holistic remedy for you, so dependence on them alone is not advisable. PE also comes with feelings of unease, despair, and hopelessness affecting your life in different ways. SSRIs, armed with serotonin, help to liven you up (Waldinger, 2007). So apart from a prolonged sexual experience, SSRIs might even give your life a little ray of sunshine.

Like many drugs, SSRIs have their ironic, albeit disappointing side effects such as a lowered libido, which some other drugs, such as Viagra, can address. One drug may not do the whole job; while it helps one thing, it also aggravates another, leaving you in need of even more drugs. Without particularly being in support of dependence on medications, I would like to say that as infuriating as it is, these drugs still do go a long way in helping you manage your condition.

Meds That May Help

Although the Food and Drug Administration in the US has not validated any medication to cure PE, below are some SSRIs that are likely to alleviate PE. The drugs are intended for other conditions but are prescribed alternatively by doctors. Doctors have no qualms prescribing these drugs because, even though like many other drugs, they have side effects. They are also relatively potent and harmless (Crenshaw & Wiesner, 1994; Montague *et al.*, 2004; Kendirci *et al.*, 2007).

Paxil (paroxetine)

- Class: SSRI

- Ideal dose: 20 milligrams per day

- Side-effects: queasiness, drowsiness, lightheadedness, parched tongue, and headache

- Directions: Should be taken daily; results may not be apparent until 3-6 weeks after the start of dose.

Men suffering from kidney and liver pathologies, coagulopathies, manic-depressive disorders, glaucoma, or someone who has had a recent cardiac arrest should not take Paxil.

N.B: There is a possibility of drug interaction with anticonvulsants (phenobarbital), anticoagulants (warfarin), alcohol, and even other antidepressants.

Prozac (fluoxetine)

- Class: SSRI

- Ideal dose: 10-20 milligram per day

- Side-effects: lightheadedness, headache, queasiness, sleeplessness, anxiety

- Directions: should be taken daily; results may not be apparent until 3-6 weeks after the start of dose

Men suffering from diabetes or epilepsy should use this drug with care.

NB: there is a possibility of drug interaction with anticonvulsants (phenobarbital), anticoagulants (warfarin), alcohol, lithium, sleeping pills, and even other antidepressants.

Zoloft (sertraline)

- Class: SSRI

- Ideal dose: 50 milligrams per day

- Side-effects: headache, sleeplessness, queasiness, diarrhea

- Directions: should be given daily; results may not be apparent until 3-6 weeks after the start of dose

Men suffering from kidney and liver pathologies, glaucoma, or someone who has had a recent cardiac arrest, should use this drug with caution.

NB: There is a possibility of drug interaction with anticoagulants (warfarin), alcohol, sleeping pills (Diazepam/Valium), and even other antidepressants.

Priligy (dapoxetine)

- Class: SSRI

- Ideal dose: 25 milligrams

- Side-effects: headache, anxiety, lightheadedness, queasiness

- Directions: not to be taken every day, but only prior to intercourse

NB: It is administered by prescription in Germany, Sweden, Finland, and some other countries. Yet to be accepted in the USA.

Viagra

- Class: Phosphodiesterase type 5 (PDE5) inhibitor

- Ideal dose: 20-50 milligrams

- Side-effects: lightheadedness, diarrhea, rhinitis, flushes, and heartburn sensations

- Directions: Not to be taken daily but just prior to intercourse

Men suffering from a recent cardiac arrest, stroke, or elevated blood pressure should use this drug with discretion. Men who also use nitrates should not use this drug.

NB: Certain interaction with nitric acids, possible interaction with some antibiotics, and protease inhibitors.

Chapter 13:

Best Positions for Lasting Longer During Sex

When you're having sex, different positions have different effects on ejaculation control. These different positions give varying levels of sensitivity and pleasure to men.

Below is a list of the best positions to last longer and improve stamina in bed during sex.

Man on Top (Missionary)

This is the most popular sex position and is usually the first one tried for many people. It's pleasurable, romantic, classic, and quite easy. While many people believe it is difficult to control arousal in this position, it is easier to control if the rate of penetration is controlled and body weight support is stronger. However, this often strains the legs and arms if not constantly practiced.

In the missionary position, you and your partner can hug, kiss, look at each other intensely in the eyes, and see each other's expressions. It is arguably the best position for intimacy. In this position, the clitoris and g-spot get some amazing stimulation. Raising up your groin a few inches and using your arms as support will increase stimulation when the woman's vulva and your pubic bone come in contact.

You'll get a deeper penetration if she opens up, and this can be achieved by gently helping her to bend her legs. You'll enjoy better leverage and control if she puts her feet below her hips and rises up using her pelvis. She can enjoy this further by grabbing your butt with her hands and pulling herself up to match your strokes. This increases her clitoral stimulation, due to the pressure angle, position intensity, and rhythmic variation.

Another way to increase the pleasure for both of you is to have her hold her legs together with your legs positioned on both sides of hers. This way, your penis will move over the clitoris during penetration.

Woman on Top (Cowgirl)

This is the second most popular sexual position. It is done with the woman on top either with her back to you or with her facing you. It is a widely accepted position by women because they can control the direction and speed of the sex.

It's a position that makes ejaculation easy to control by men. This is because, being on your back relaxes you and allows you to concentrate on and become aware of your arousal state, breathing patterns, PC muscles, speed, and motion.

Depending on your goals and needs, this position can be altered a bit for an amazing effect. Different results can be achieved from slightly realigning your legs or hips, or going faster or slower. Try out different alterations for this position to see how it helps you to have better in-bed stamina and a more enjoyable experience for you and your partner.

Doggy Style

The doggy style position, in many lovers' opinions, gives the utmost pleasure to both women and men. It is related to animalism and instinct. It gives me the feeling of being dominant, while women get the feeling of being 'taken.' Also from a psychological point of view, this position represents an archaic model in which the human being sees life, that is, the woman first of all and the man behind him ready to protect it.

It allows for deeper penetration and intense stimulation of the g-spot.

In this position, ease the pressure off your legs by standing at the edge of the bed or kneeling on the bed, rather than squatting.

In this style, the woman kneels, pushing up her backside, helping her to naturally open up slightly more allowing for the penis to penetrate deeper. The deep penetration of the penis reduces stimulation on the penis head, helping you to control orgasm and last longer.

A slight variation to this position can be for your partner to lie flat on her belly with you on top of her, coming in from behind. This helps your bodies to be closer to each other in their entirety, leading to a more physical and verbal intimacy between you both.

Side by Side

The side-by-side technique is commonly called 'spooning,' and is a useful position to make you last longer during sex. It's the best position for when you have morning sex, when you feel tired, and if you have any physical limitations, such as a back problem. Due to the heavy kissing and tight hugging possible in this position, the height of intimacy can skyrocket.

To enjoy it better, intertwine or 'scissor' you and your partner's legs. It realigns your angle and position, as well as shifts weight in such a way that you now have full control in the process.

Standing

The standing technique is a considered a less traditional sex position. The fun thing about this position is that you can do it at any safe place if you're taken in the moment. However, due to differences in angles and height, difficulties can arise.

The best way to enjoy control over your arousal state in this position is to prop against a table or wall, experimenting with different leg positions and angles until you arrive at a suitable position for both of you. With you in control, you can become aware of your ejaculation timing.

Chapter 14:

Extra Tips to Overcome Premature Ejaculation

Patience

The journey will not be all rainbows and sunshine but with commitment, persistence, and patience, you will pull it off. There is no cure for PE. You will need to combine medications and exercises. The exercises will take time to see results. However, if you stick to your carefully planned routine, then you can enjoy an improved sex life too. You will make more than a few errors, but if you keep at getting it right, you will succeed.

Be relentless! Management for a chronic condition like PE will need a box of life tools to combat your PE. In addition to medications and exercises, you need an optimistic mental outlook. You already have all the tools from this book Use them! I can assure you that you will get through this, and you can enjoy sex with your partner with gratifying orgasms.

Don't overexert yourself. Go at your own pace to avoid anxiety and nervous wrecks. Look towards the years of bliss you will have ahead of you, and don't let these few months of trials and errors get to you.

Visualization

Having an optimistic outlook plays a substantial part in the outcome and satisfaction you develop when overcoming any obstacle. By erasing the negative aura and effect of the shame associated with premature ejaculation, you will discover sex to be more pleasing and perform longer than expected.

Irrespective of how you are feeling: take a moment, remove from your mind the word *impossible*, and instead focus your mind and energy on what is possible.

Always reassure yourself that you can take charge of your inner strength. You can perform for a prolonged time in bed and slow down orgasm according to your time frame. Declare it continually, and you will begin to accept it as the truth. Your lasting power will begin to improve, and it will boost your sexual prowess.Declare to yourself continually that YOU can, and your IO will begin to accept it as an absolute truth. This is called neuro-linguistic programming (NLP). Your enduring power will begin to improve, and your sexual prowess will increase.

Merged with visualization techniques, such as visualizing yourself experiencing pleasurable sex can help your approach to sex. If it's a complicated position that makes you orgasm faster, conjure images in your mind of having sex in that position for a prolonged period.

If you find your partner's physical appearance to be alluring, visualize you are together (or other women that you find enticing) frequently. To make the experience more accurate, you need to visualize the whole experience from meeting a girl to talking to dancing to kissing to smooching and finally to sex. Go into the specifics. Own it and visualize it. Fantasize what it would feel like being inside your partner, and all the feelings, smells, tastes, and pleasures that go along with it.

To make the experience pleasurable and satisfying, it is not helpful to feel uneasy. Imagine yourself getting it right and even picture the inhalation and exhalation technique we discussed earlier. Imagine feeling relaxed and breathing normally, but not yet blown away by the good sex. This establishes a yardstick to distance yourself and convinces you that you have experienced it in the past. It gives you the impression that it has occurred before and you can do it again. Rehearse this daily for about 5-10 minutes, and you can anticipate and influence the actual bedroom outcome.

Exceptional minds and talented athletes value the importance of visualization and how functional the mind can be when utilizing energy to yield remarkable results. Visualization techniques also take time and patience. It is important to move forward with continual effort and practice.

Masturbation Before Sex

If masturbation is useful for premature ejaculation, does it mean you should masturbate before sex? This is a technique that men with premature ejaculation have exhausted thinking you should masturbate now to "get it off your mind," so you can perform longer during actual sex.

Quite sadly, it is not as easy as masturbating before sex to slow down ejaculation. It is a temporary fix, not a logical long-term approach. In my observation, older men find it hard to retain an erection once they have masturbated, while young men find it easy to retain an erection during actual sex and their IELT does not increase.

Few men have realized that they are able to retain mild erection and still ejaculate after a short while. It is possible for a man to ejaculate without getting an erection, and most men with premature ejaculation have experienced this. If it eventually works, masturbating before sex only hides the reality that you have premature ejaculation, it doesn't solve the real issue.

Sex is a Game, Have Fun.

If you pause and reflect on sex for a second, you will probably realize that God has a very good sense of humor.

Possessing a very good sense of humor about sex helps in times when things don't flow as you want: you can't change positions, someone gets hurt as a result of the other person moving, your body makes a disgusting noise, or one of you utters a nonsensical statement right before or after orgasm.

A sense of playfulness is a very good thing to bring to bed.

From the first hint to foreplay to the last sigh, everything about sex should be fun. Tease one another and be silly. Enjoy one another and allow things to head where they will. Rid yourselves of the fear of what may or may not happen and experiment new things.

If the fun in your sex life has died down, reignite it again. Test boundaries in a casual and light-hearted manner, encourage and motivate her to do likewise. Remove the pressure of sex and turn it into something you both enjoy beyond the normal pleasure of orgasm.

Men very often might be ready for sex at any time, but women generally need to mentally prepare first. Try to sit down and spell out which nights you are both free to spend some quality sensual time together. Plan on a date night once a week to kick off your new playful sexual lives.

If you can't go out wait until the children are tucked in, and turn these moments into your own special time. Forget about whatever duty that needs to be attended to. Have a glass of wine, play and dance to some nice romantic music, and have a good time before retiring to the bedroom. Turn your bedroom to an intimate space with soft and romantic lighting, candles, beautiful sheets, no television, and don't forget to put a lock on the door!

Turn every chance at sex into an enjoyable and fun-filled one. It will more likely be explosive and enjoyable in the ways you can hardly imagine. It transforms every sex occasion into a pleasant and amusing occasion and not just a simple physical necessity to give vent to.

Daily Ritual

One of your best investments in learning ejaculation control will be developing a daily plan for yourself. This daily plan doesn't have to take longer than 30 minutes per day. The exercises in this book are enough for you to overcome PE.

Draw out a six-day per week plan for yourself and aim at reaching multi-orgasm, without ejaculating (if possible). Work towards ejaculating only once per week. It is normal to find people who believe that orgasm and ejaculation are the same thing because they occur simultaneously. However, with constant exercise, you can have multiple orgasms and not ejaculate.

It can take some men longer than one month to attain this goal, others less. Regardless of how long it takes, it'll be worth the work and wait.

The common phenomenon is to have sex, reach orgasm, ejaculate, feel tired, and sleep. However, you'll enjoy it more if you can have multiple orgasms without ejaculating.

Day one

- Kegel Exercise – 20 minutes

- Breathing Exercise - 10 minutes

Day two

- Meditation – 20 minutes

- Squeeze technique – 10 minutes

These are possible combinations of the exercises discussed in previous chapters. Make your own mix and match based on personal preferences and state of mind, but try to create a balance between all exercises.

Delaying Your Orgasm

The strategies mentioned earlier in this book will point you in the right direction when it comes to improving your sexual stamina, but there are still a few more strategies that can be used to prolong your orgasm while you are practicing and getting used to these exercises.

Your first choice is to use a condom during every sexual encounter you have. For apparent reasons, this is safer and it also numbs your penis and prolongs sex. They are easily available and will help to prolong the length of your sexual relations.

Secondly, select a style and master it. This book has explained the best orgasm delaying styles, and there are individual variations in the effectiveness of these styles. So, it is advisable that you select something that is effective for you and the situation you are in. Begin with it and follow through.

Reflecting on the masturbation strategies we discussed previously, if the slow technique helped you last longer, then practice that in your bedroom and do the same for the withdrawal technique. Also, just a while before reaching orgasm, pull out and reduce the pace of your thrusts.

Keep in mind to control your breathing and deploy the strategies that were mentioned in the breathing chapter of this book.

If your lover is interested, normalize the atmosphere by engaging in a light conversation. This distraction technique can help to eliminate the pressure to ejaculate and it distracts your mind from arousal.

Another strategy to delay your PE is to practice thrust control when you are close to ejaculation and you can do this by becoming attentive to the period when you are almost there, decrease the pace of your thrusts or completely penetrate your partner without thrusting to decrease your excitement levels. Remaining in there, without action, is not something so absurd. You can consider it as another form that you have to enjoy and feel your partner, try to capture its temperature, its internal dimensions, try to listen to its micro convulsions. Personally I think this is a technique that gives a lot of intimacy to the couple. Yes, because many times, as mentioned above, we take too much care to do and not to hear. You also allow her to notice and enjoy your presence. Remember, there's no hurry.

It makes no difference whether you are doing the doggy position, the in and out position in missionary, or maybe she is on top and moving up and down. As soon as you become aware that you are getting more excited, put a stop to the thrusts. Keep in mind that this should happen before you are about to reach orgasm.

This can help you move backwards and forwards. Make a few thrusts, then rest and make minimal movement. Make another thrust and stop. The deeper your penetration, the lower the level of arousal. An added bonus is that a lot of women enjoy sex using this method.

It might also be beneficial to periodically change positions. This is because the consistent motions and periods of rest reduce the levels of excitement. Undoubtedly, women have no problems with this because it spices things up and makes you come across as a dominant and self-confident.

To refresh your woman while keeping the levels of excitement, you can switch from penetrative sex to oral sex. There is no shortage of methods of adjusting or stopping sex to restore your excitement and thus allowing you to continue the sexual experience feeling revived and ready for more.

Now that you have a few ideas, you can put everything together and merge all of these strategies in any order you like. For instance, you can begin at the end by engaging in a light conversation. Then engage in foreplay and playfully pace your thrust during sex.

When you appear self-confident and make her think you are in total control of your PE, she will love it. These methods will get that message across. After a while, you will both notice an improvement in your skill and the duration of your sexual encounters. Eventually, lasting during sex will come naturally to you and you will be able to do without these methods and tricks like second nature.

Your Ideal Partner

It is also helpful to highlight the features of a woman who is generally compatible with a man with PE.

- She doesn't mind other means of sexual gratification and orgasms such as orally or by hand.

- She is honest about her sexual excitement and doesn't pretend to climax.

- She says what she means and means what she says. When she isn't happy about a situation, she won't lie about it.

- She must be tolerant and understanding. This is because the man with PE will need to have a routine for sex, which could end up being boring and monotonous.

- She is aware that your PE is a medical condition and not an indication of your interest in her or of a lack of sensitivity towards her needs.

- Does not particularly require a lot of work (for the release of dopamine) in order to be sexually aroused.

- Is tolerant of your tendency to climax too soon.

- She is content with having as many orgasms as you can give her, not particularly concurrently.

- Is open with you on the topic of your PE.

Perhaps the most important of these characteristics is her ability to talk freely with you about your condition, even if she doesn't have all the other features. As long as she is open, don't be worried. She will learn to adapt to the situation and adjust her sexual expectations. With her understanding and openness, you can both grow your relationship.

Conclusion

The majority of men prefer to remain in their comfort zone, reluctant to take full control of their sex lives, not bold enough to break the cycle of premature ejaculation. Some are not even convinced that it is possible to defeat it while some are also of the opinion that "it's too much effort".

Luckily, you have refused to be one of them. Instead, you have plucked up courage by identifying the issue causing you distress and decided to deal with it. You, my friend, are a FIXER who takes pride in gaining control of his life, not a grumbler. We are alike, and it is my wish to share how I overcame it, so other men can learn from my experience. The information provided above is from experience. Remember the importance of mind and body in defeating PE. We are what we conceive in our mind. Our ideas mold our feelings and our feelings mold our lives.

False ideas and false presumptions will eventually lead to cynical perceptions of sex. Your mind could either serve as your greatest weapon or your worst enemy. It solely lies on what you feed it. The majority of men suffering from premature ejaculation all lack the idea of what good sex is. They are of the opinion that good sex is a strenuous sport that ought to take place for hours. They view their partner's orgasm as one of their consecrated task and responsibility. Eventually, it causes them to experience sex not as their own masculine pleasure but as an avenue to show themselves worthy.

This will lead to ingrained pressure on your sex life and can result in an opposite effect. Say goodbye to wrong ideas and myths.

Try to position your thinking to affect how you perceive

yourself, sex, and women. The faster you discard negative thoughts; the faster the premature ejaculation begins to fade away.

Nonetheless, perception is not the only thing men with premature ejaculation have in common. They also lack the realization of their primary body functions. Rehearse acquiring power over your breathing and muscles. Learn to feel anxiety and calm down willingly. Learn to gain control over how you get aroused sexually and ejaculate.

This book has been designed to help you perform longer in bed. But even more than that, it can be utilized to increase your general sexual desires and serve as a support to your relationship through intimacy and communication. Begin some of the training and be assured that if you follow the information, you are on the ladder towards sexual gratification and fulfillment.

The ball now lies in your court; you have all the necessary information. You now have the power to join the league of men.

References

Alghobary, M., El-Bayoumy, Y., Mostafa, Y., Mahmoud, E. H. M., & Amr, M. (2010). Evaluation of tramadol on demand vs. Daily paroxetine as a long-term treatment of lifelong premature ejaculation. *The journal of sexual medicine*, *7*(8), 2860-2867.

Althof, S. E. (2005). Psychological treatment strategies for rapid ejaculation: rationale, practical aspects, and outcome. *World journal of urology*, *23*(2), 89-92.

Althof, S. E., & McMahon, C. G. (2016). Contemporary management of disorders of male orgasm and ejaculation. *Urology*, *93*, 9-21.

Ashburn, T. T., & Thor, K. B. (2004). Drug repositioning: identifying and developing new uses for existing drugs. *Nature reviews Drug discovery*, *3*(8), 673.

Betchen, S. J. (2015). Premature Ejaculation: An Integrative, Intersystems Approach for Couples. In *Systemic sex therapy*(pp. 122-138). Routledge.

Buffum, J. (1986). Pharmacosexology update: prescription drugs and sexual function. *Journal of psychoactive drugs*, *18*(2), 97-106.

Cavallini, G., & Maretti, C. (2017). Relationship between the Wording of the Instructions and the Efficacy of Dapoxetine in the Therapy of Lifelong Premature Ejaculation: A Pilot Study. *Global Journal of Medical Research*.

Ciocca, G., Limoncin, E., Mollaioli, D., Gravina, G. L., Di Sante, S., Carosa, E., ... & Jannini, E. A. (2013). Integrating psychotherapy and pharmacotherapy in the treatment of premature ejaculation. *Arab journal of urology, 11*(3), 305-312.

Crenshaw, R. T., & Wiesner, M. G. (1994). U.S. Patent No. 5,276,042. Washington, DC: U.S. Patent and Trademark Office.

Dhikav, V., Karmarkar, G., Gupta, M., & Anand, K. (2007). ORIGINAL RESEARCH—EJACULATORY DISORDERS: Yoga in Premature Ejaculation: A Comparative Trial with Fluoxetine. The Journal Of Sexual Medicine, 4(6), 1726-1732. doi: 10.1111/j.1743-6109.2007.00603.x

Giami, A., Laumann, E., Gagnon, J., Michael, R., Michaels, S., & Michael, R. et al. (1997). The Social Organization of Sexuality. Sexual Practices in the United States. *Population (French Edition), 52*(6), 1548. doi: 10.2307/1534637

Godman, H. (2019). Erectile Dysfunction (ED): Causes, Treatment, and More. Retrieved 5 July 2019, from https://www.healthline.com/health/erectile-dysfunction

Gur, S., & Sikka, S. C. (2015). The characterization, current medications, and promising therapeutics targets for premature ejaculation. *Andrology, 3*(3), 424-442.

Harvey, K. Y., & Balon, R. (1995). Clinical implications of antidepressant drug effects on sexual function. *Annals of clinical psychiatry, 7*(4), 189-200.

ISSM. (2019). Definition of Premature Ejaculation (PE) | ISSM. Retrieved 6 July 2019, from https://www.issm.info/news/sex-health-headlines/definition-of-premature-ejaculation-pe/

Jain, A. (2017). Yoga asanas That can cure Premature Ejaculation. Retrieved 5 July 2019, from https://www.drakjainclinic.com/yoga-asanas-can-cure-premature-ejaculation/

Kaplan, H. S., Kohl, R. N., Pomeroy, W. B., Offit, A. K., & Hogan, B. (1974). Group treatment of premature ejaculation. *Archives of Sexual Behavior*, *3*(5), 443-452.

Kendirci, M., Salem, E., & Hellstrom, W. J. (2007). Dapoxetine, a novel selective serotonin transport inhibitor for the treatment of premature ejaculation. Therapeutics and clinical risk management, 3(2), 277.

Leiblum, S. R., & Rosen, R. C. (Eds.). (1989). Principles and practice of sex therapy: Update for the 1990s (2nd ed.). New York, NY, US: Guilford Press.

Mamidi, P., & Gupta, K. (2013). Efficacy of certain yogic and naturopathic procedures in premature ejaculation: A pilot study. International Journal Of Yoga, 6(2), 118. doi: 10.4103/0973-6131.113408

McMahon, C. G. (2008). Clinical trial methodology in premature ejaculation observational, interventional, and treatment preference studies—Part I—Defining and selecting the study population. *The journal of sexual medicine*, *5*(8), 1805-1816.

Montague, D. K., Jarow, J., Broderick, G. A., Dmochowski, R. R., Heaton, J. P., Lue, T. F., ... & AUA Erectile Dysfunction Guideline Update Panel. (2004). AUA guideline on the pharmacologic management of premature ejaculation. The Journal of urology, 172(1), 290-294.

Porst, H., Montorsi, F., Rosen, R. C., Gaynor, L., Grupe, S., & Alexander, J. (2007). The Premature Ejaculation Prevalence and Attitudes (PEPA) survey: prevalence, comorbidities, and professional help-seeking. *European urology, 51*(3), 816-824.

Rosen, R. C. (2001). Psychogenic erectile dysfunction: classification and management. *Urologic Clinics of North America, 28*(2), 269-278.

Salonia, A., Saccà, A., Briganti, A., Del Carro, U., Dehò, F., & Zanni, G. et al. (2009). Original Research—Ejaculatory Disorders: Quantitative Sensory Testing of Peripheral Thresholds in Patients with Lifelong Premature Ejaculation: A Case-Controlled Study. *The Journal Of Sexual Medicine, 6*(6), 1755-1762. doi: 10.1111/j.1743-6109.2009.01276.x

Seo, D. H., Jeh, S. U., Choi, S. M., Kam, S. C., Kim, S. W., Yang, D. Y., ... & Hyun, J. S. (2016). Diagnosis and treatment of premature ejaculation by urologists in South Korea. *The world journal of men's health, 34*(3), 217-223.

Smalley, G. (2018). Men and Intimacy - iMom. Retrieved 7 July 2019, from https://www.imom.com/men-and-intimacy/#.XTHXIypDDMU

The Health Site. (2014). Yoga pose for a stronger orgasm -- Dhanurasana | TheHealthSite.com. Retrieved 9 July 2019, from https://www.thehealthsite.com/fitness/yoga/yoga-pose-for-a-stronger-orgasm-dhanurasana-p114-115837/

The Health Site. (2015). Yoga to beat premature ejaculation and last longer during sex. Retrieved 6 July 2019, from https://www.thehealthsite.com/fitness/yoga/control-premature-ejaculation-with-yoga-p114-114625/

Waldinger, M. D., Schweitzer, D. H., & Olivier, B. (2005). On-demand SSRI treatment of premature ejaculation: pharmacodynamic limitations for relevant ejaculation delay and consequent solutions. The journal of sexual medicine